# a Better Way

# a Better Way

## Your guide to abundant health

Dr. Jody Cox, D.C.

Revised July 2018.

Cover Art: Rebecca Siewert of Rebecca Siewert Photography

Disclaimer

This book has been written strictly for educational and informational purposes. It is not intended to serve as medical treatment or as medical advice. This book is not intended to diagnose or treat any medical condition. Using any of the information in this book is based on the reader's own judgement after consulting with his or her physician or other medical practitioner.

Published by Prominence Publishing, www.prominencepublishing.com

To connect with Dr. Jody Cox, visit www.DrJodyCox.com

# Foreword

Life can be compared to a marathon that we need to run with perseverance and train for properly.

Years ago I taught a 2-day course to a group of women who were business leaders in my city about taking charge and being good stewards of their health. We talked about everything from spinal health to nutrition, exercise to sleep, from anti-aging (and aging gracefully) to brain health. One of the underlying premises was that we have only one body and one life, and the choices we make today not only affect, but *become* our bodies tomorrow.

Making good choices and sticking to them is much more difficult than it seems. The confusing world surrounding how we handle our health - from what we eat, to how we exercise, to our healthcare choices - are swamped in a plethora of options and conflicting opinions.

**One of your most vital and essential jobs on this earth is to steward your body properly.** If you aren't healthy, strong and clear-minded, how will you take care of every other important job and opportunity that you are given? Most people take better care of their *cars* then they do their own body. Making the right choices and then training hard within them is the key to success.

1Corinthians 3:16 states "Don't you know that you yourselves are God's temple, and that God's Spirit lives in you?"

As a primary health care provider who has been in the business for over 25 years and as a mother and coach, I have seen the tide of opinion sway from one extreme to the other and back again. I've witnessed the aisles of our grocery stores fill up with products that were only available in obscure health food stores just 10-15 years ago.

In healthcare, we talk a lot about informed consent. Legally, ethically, and just plain intelligently, it is a wise move to investigate your options and then make the best informed choice.

**A Better Way** will answer important questions about your choices for optimal health and how to integrate all of it for a healthy family. Dr. Jody's positive, high energy, and sometimes 'just plain crazy' zeal for health and approach to life is as infectious as it is effective.

I suggest you 'shut down, sit up and listen' to what she is offering you here in **A Better Way.** Without a plan, you will end up someplace else and in the wrong body. **You just need to begin**.

Step out of your comfort zone and train in a different one. You won't change or see the results you are looking for until you do.

Marie T Geschwandtner,
DC Head Women's Coach,
Warrior Coaching Principle,
Chiropractors With Compassion Ottawa, Ontario

# Dedication

This book is dedicated to my biological children Clara and Ian; and my Compassion children: Samuel, Jennifer and Yumari. They are so patient, forgiving, and loveable. They keep me in a state of awe and constantly remind me to laugh and dream.

They are already becoming World Changers. This is one of my legacy gifts to them.

# Contents

# Acknowledgments

It goes without saying, but I am of the thousands of chiropractors along this continuum of chiropractic. I am honored and privileged to be in such a great and noble profession. Back in the early 1900's, there were only a handful of chiropractors that brought forth chiropractic and planted the seeds for the generations to come. They were the outcasts and looked like radicals at their time because Chiropractic was not acknowledged as mainstream yet. I am so grateful for their fearless passion and sacrifices to preserve chiropractic. It is because of these people who pursued the truth and followed their dreams, that I have a better life, and you will too.

Many other amazing mentors have personally helped me flourish in my career along the way and have provided much of the inspiration for the contents of this book including my friends at Warrior Coaching; my Chiropractic pals at The Holding Tank; my book coach, Suzanne Doyle-Ingram of Prominence Publishing; and without exception, my friend and devoted husband, Dr. Ron Pashkewych, who has patiently and lovingly walked through this journey with me every step of the way.

Of course, nothing would be anything if not for my Savior Jesus Christ; who gets all the glory - especially if this book inspires you or changes you in any way.

# Introduction

This book is not a quick fix.

There is no magic pill nor secrets here.

This book is about true health, and how YOU can experience life fully alive

—For the rest of your life!

This is not a pile of information. You've got enough already. We live in a world where we have everything accessible at our fingertips. You can Google just about anything to find what you are looking for, and obtain it instantly. With so much accessibility to everything you need or have already, why would you need this book?

My guess is if you are like me, you need a straight clear path away through all the confusion of mixed messages on what you should and shouldn't do when it comes to your health. You are the type who wants the best for your family and are hoping to find solutions based on solid truth while not being manipulated with fear. The pressure to get onboard with the 'next best trendy thing' is exhausting you. I'm also guessing that you don't want to settle for being told, that when it comes to your state of health, that "this is as good as it gets".

You might be the person who is already living the dream, but deep down inside you know that sooner or later, your negated health habits – albeit physically or emotionally, will catch up to you, and before an inevitable crisis occurs, you need some redirection to get you on the right track - now. Essentially, this book is a reboot for you.

Regardless of where you are in your life's journey, this book will be a lighthouse for you and will point the way so that you can truly live a higher quality of life.

But before you go on, you need to ask yourself one question:

"WHY?"

Why do you want to be healthy?

Because what you are going to learn and discover throughout this book has the power to literally transform your life and the life of your family. But here's the catch: This book and all the tools and tips in it will not change your life unless you start thinking about "the Big Why?"

## WHY DO YOU WANT TO HAVE ABUNDANT HEALTH?

Take a moment to ponder that question.

Once you get a glimpse of your "WHY", then dive into this book. Your WHY will be the anchor in your transformation.

My hope for you is that you find answers to your questions and bring clarity for your health goals, as well as amplify the vision for your life.

And then the fun part begins--when you take action.

Lastly, you may hear numerous times that I mention "God" throughout this book. Trust me, this is not a Christian self-help book where you are going to feel offended or condemned if you don't believe in God. I am only sharing my belief, and would be a hypocrite if I didn't give credit where credit is due. But don't let my spiritual belief get in the way from you fully learning everything this book has to offer which is based on years of science, research and expertise—all pointing to simply a better way.

# PART ONE:

## A Better Way to Health

# Chapter 1: How Do You Know If You Are Healthy?

*True health comes from within, or in other words: 'Smiling on the inside'.*

If you were asked, "How do you know if you are healthy?" What would you say?

"I'm healthy because I feel good." Right?

Let's think about that. Have you heard of someone you thought was 'healthy' and then you suddenly find out that they had a heart attack? Before they had that heart attack, you thought they were perfectly healthy though. What does that mean?

See, if you base your health strictly on how you are 'feeling' or looking, you could be missing a vital key to understanding true health.

Everything you are about to discover in this section is going to show you and your family how to BE truly healthy. In other words, "smiling on the inside". You are about to learn the truth about where health comes from and how to stay healthy and enjoy your life-fully. This book is meant to challenge you. But I promise that if you can apply some of the truths and principles given, it can not only potentially save your life, but also lead you and your family towards living a higher quality of life. That is my hope for you.

*Our story begins with a young mom named Anne, who had big dreams to be an interior designer but is currently working part-time as a receptionist at the library. She has two adorable children in elementary school and has been married to Craig for 7 years, who is a full-time computer programmer. She lives in a modest home and a nice neighborhood.*

*Unfortunately, even though everything appears to be great, Anne is not. In fact, she has been suffering from daily headaches and low-grade anxiety over the past 5 years. She has tight shoulders, and periodic digestive problems. With the demands of running the home, work, and kids' activities, she finds little time for herself.*

*Finally, Anne sought out her family doctor because she desperately needed relief. He took a health history, listened to her symptoms, and prescribed Celebrex to help with her headaches and tight shoulders. She gratefully took the medication and noticed a change immediately, and within a few days, felt like she was back to her normal self.*

*However, a few weeks went by and the headaches slowly started to come back again.*

*In addition, she started experiencing more constipation and bloating. She called her family doctor and this time he suggested that she double the dose of her medication. She took his advice and for a few more days everything seemed to work but once again the headaches came back, stronger than ever. Now she was beginning to experience a burning sensation every time she ate. One of her friends suggested to her that she try taking some Tums to give her relief. She once again consulted* her doctor and now was prescribed another pain medication and referred her for a CT scan. She was also prescribed an antacid to help combat the burning sensation in her stomach and take a daily Metamucil to help resolve the constipation. The CT scan came back negative, but her symptoms still persisted.

A few years went by and Anne was just learning to live with it all. She continued to take her daily headache medication and added a few Tylenol 3s every couple of days to help her cope. The Tums and Metamucil were now a regular part of her daily routine to counterbalance her digestive issues.

With the new stresses of her husband's job loss and the demands of her growing children's extra activities, she started experiencing fatigue more often. The more tired she got, the more coffee she needed. And when coffee didn't kick it, she would reach for a Diet Coke to help carry her through. And at the end of the day when she found it all too overwhelming, she found that a few glasses of wine, chips and a candy bar would be great to 'take the edge off' and help get through the final two hours of the evening.

Flash forward to the present day, and now she finds herself waking up stiff and achy. She can't seem to think or focus clearly on things anymore and feels like she is in a mental fog. She has also gained some weight due to her late night indulgences. She can't understand why this has happened to her, but it doesn't really matter. She has convinced herself that this is as good as it gets. She has a bathroom cabinet full of different prescriptions to put out whatever pain comes her way. She is barely coping. She starts experiencing bouts of melancholy, which eventually turned into bigger bouts of anxiety and depression.

*She visits her doctor who decides that perhaps she should try an antidepressant to help her get through this tough time and help keep her going. And even though she doesn't want to, she figures that it might be what she needs at this time - after all, she has tried everything. And at least this will help her so she can get through life; after all, as her mother reminds her, "You are getting older".*

Is this how life is supposed to be?

What happened to her health?

What happened to her dreams?

What will happen to the future of her kids? Will they experience the same pattern of needlessly silently suffering?

Is all hope lost?

I don't know if you can relate to some of this or all of this, but this is a story about how you can one day out of nowhere wake up and realize that the life you were hoping for is far from your reality. The truth is, this is a real story. And Anne (name changed) is not the only one. I know there are hundreds of 'Anne's' out there because stories like this are common when people first come into my practice. And I'm here to tell you two things:

1.   Life is about living Fully Alive – in ALL things. and

2.   Your story can be So

# Much

# Better!

To understand how to live a life fully alive, stay focused-- so that by the end of this book, you will be fully equipped on how to live in abundant health, make better decisions for you and your family, go after your dreams, and finally experience a deep peace and joy throughout the process.

The first thing you need to know is that:

You are created to be *fully* alive and live out your purpose here on earth. You are not designed to be sick or dis-eased.

*"You are designed to be healthy*
*and heal yourself"*

# Chapter 2: Where Does Your Health Come From?

Have you ever wondered how some people have abundant health and it seems so effortless? They just seem to be glowing, fit, balanced, energized and joyful? And when you get to know them, you realize they are authentic and congruent in their healthy lifestyle.

Did they get there by random chance?

Or do they just have good luck?

Or good genes?

Nope.

They have simply made better choices all along the way.

## ARE WE MACHINES?

It is all about choices--the gift of free will. And once you begin to understand your health care choices and options, you will be able to make wiser decisions for you and your family. It starts with understanding the two main dominant models of health care that we utilize in our society. One is overtly dominant, and is called the 'Mechanistic" model of care, and the other is called the 'Vitalistic' model of care. Both models are extremely valuable and applicable. But what has happened is that society has adapted one model to the extreme, which is causing us a lot of problems.

Let's start off with the Mechanistic model of care. In the mechanistic model, the underlying philosophy is that you and I are a bunch of mechanical parts and we can't fix ourselves. Being healthy or sick is a random chance, and there is little to no acknowledgment that your body can heal itself.

In that model, you are viewed as a machine. For example, let's say, you have a car, and it is broken down, and you have it towed to your driveway, and you leave it there. Is there any expectation that it will restore itself on its own? No. In fact, if you just leave it there, it will eventually rot and rust.

Now let's apply this model to you. Let's say your body is broken down and you got back pain, or some digestive issues, or even arm numbness. Essentially you have 'DIS--EASE'. As a result, you head to the Doctor's office, because that is what most people do as their first line of defense. If you go see a Doctor, who works in that Mechanistic model (and not all doctors do) who gives little to no acknowledgment that your body can fix itself, he or she will have to give you something from the outside to fix the inside. So 90% of the time you are going to leave the doctor's office with what? I'm guessing drugs or a prescription. And here lies the problem: The mechanistic model addresses the **symptoms** and not the **cause.**

So if you have a headache, or your digestion is malfunctioning, or you have a pain going down your leg, and you take an Advil for that---is pill going to address the *cause* of the problem? What if you take a muscle relaxant, is that going to address the cause of the problem? Those drugs are addressing the symptoms, but not the true cause.

And it gets worse than that because what happens if that drug actually starts working, and takes away all your symptoms? You start thinking you are totally better. But in reality, all it is doing is just masking the problem inside, quieting the symptoms, and meanwhile all this time your body is continuing to break down because the *cause* of the problem was never addressed.

So the drugs are addressing the symptoms and not the cause. Just so you know, we are not anti-drug nor anti-medical. The Mechanistic system was actually designed and created for crisis and trauma. Which means, if you needed a quadruple bypass because your lifestyle has been terrible for the last 30 years, or you have bad genes (and you can blame your parents for that), it is amazing that we have the Heart Institute and talented surgeons who can perform a quadruple bypass surgery and save your life. Or what if you have a child at home and they are fatally ill and there is an antibiotic you can give them to save their life? That would be crisis. Would you believe that is a good thing? Absolutely. So the model works for crisis, and it also works for trauma.

If I were to run across the highway without looking and I got run over by a car and had body parts all over the place, a hospital is where I need to go. There, the emergency doctors can sew me back up, pump me full of drugs and try to save my life. That's a good place to be, and we all should be so grateful that we have a place with these skilled people who can take care of us should crisis or trauma ever happen. In these cases, the Mechanistic model of health is very applicable and important.

But you can't take a model that is based on disease, meaning we wait for the symptoms to be there, and then try and fix it with drugs and surgery and call it health. So how are we doing in?

What is the leading cause of death in Canada? Cancer. In fact, it is expected that 2 out of every 5 Canadians will develop cancer in their lifetime. Each hour, it is estimated that 21 people will be diagnosed with cancer in Canada1, and one person dies from cancer every 17 minutes.2 So by the time you finish reading this book in approximately 5 hours, about 100 people in our country will have been told they have cancer and 17 people will have died.

Heart Disease is the second leading cause of death in Canada. Moe than 1.37 million Canadians have heart disease. It is also one of the leading causes of death in Canada[3], claiming the death of a person every 14 minutes.[4]

The 3rd leading cause of death might surprise you. It is reactions to drugs and medical error![5] It is actually published in the Journal of the American Medical Association. Statistically, it is suggested that about 40,000 serious adverse drug reactions occur annually in Canada, even when the person is taking the right prescribed drug for the right reason.[6]

In Canadian hospitals, according to the Canadian Medical Association Journal in 2004, adverse events occur in 7.5% of patients.[7] Recent studies have shown that adverse event rate to have increased to 10-14%[8]

Johns Hopkins Medical School refined this research and discovered that medical errors and prescription drugs together may actually be the LEADING cause of death and are responsible for 400,000 deaths per year.[9]

So you've got to ask yourself, "How are we doing?" Not so good? And typically what are your choices under that mechanistic model as a solution if you do get cancer or heart disease?

Now, this information is not to discourage you, but to get you thinking. Because this is not the end of the story. There are other options.

There is definitely a better way.

## HEALTHY BY DESIGN

As far as healthcare goes, if you are going to not only just survive but actually thrive in your health, then you need to embrace the Vitalistic Model of Health Care. The premise of this model is really simple. The Vitalistic model of health suggests that you and I have an innate power within us that runs our bodies. Our bodies were designed specially to heal from the inside out without the use of drugs and surgery most of the time, except in extreme situations of crisis and trauma. That's pretty different than the Mechanistic model which looks at your body as a machine which cannot fix itself. Did you ever wonder how a cut on your hand heals so perfectly that weeks later, you can't see where that cut actually was? Or if you ever broke a bone, your body somehow knows how to re-connect the bone and heal it? Have you ever had the flu and after a few days of fever, chills and generally feeling lousy you fully recover? There is a power inside you that works to repair, function, and recreate within your body. You were born with it. You and I are designed to be healthy, purposeful human beings living fully alive for 90-110 years. Your body has a power inside itself that allows you to heal from above - down – inside - out.

There is an internal intelligence that guides this perfect process. People have different ideas about what to call this intelligence, and even different ideas about where it came from in the first place. For me, I believe that God breathes that life into us.[10][11][12] Some call it Mother Nature. The Chinese call this power chi, and Indian culture calls it prana. I have heard it be called the life force or the vital force. Chiropractors call it innate intelligence. For the purposes of simplicity, I'll just call it LIFE. Regardless of what you call it, we need to recognize that there is an intelligence that runs our body whose power exceeds our understanding. Let me prove that to you:

There isn't a single surgeon on the planet who would do surgery on anybody without knowing this basic healing principle; after the surgery has been completed and the tissues are approximated and are stitched up, the doctor is free to go home even while you are still in the hospital bed. Why is this possible? The reason is because at this point you begin the healing process. Your healing power is working.

If I was to cut my hand right now, instantly hundreds of processes happen so that my body begins the healing process. Do you need to think about it? No. It just happens and it happens perfectly every time.


## YOU ARE TRULY A MIRACLE

Here is a final illustration of that magnificent power within you.

Have you ever wondered how you were formed? In a nutshell, at conception, two half cells (sperm and an egg) are united and create one cell. Then that one cell begins to divide. Days later, there are hundreds of thousands of cells and they were all identical. They were not differentiated - they all looked exactly the same.

Twenty-one days after conception a brain and spinal cord-a rudimentary nervous system began to develop.

The nervous system orchestrates the development of the rest

of your body. At this time, your cells began to differentiate. The brain and nervous system say "Ok, you're going to be a kidney cell, and you're going to go over here, and you're going to be a liver cell, and you're going to go here and you're going to be a red blood cell, and a white blood cell, and a nerve cell, and a muscle cell, a tissue cell, etc." You get the picture....

Nine months later, there are nine trillion cells, the organ systems are functioning perfectly and the result is about 7 pounds and 10 inches (give or take) of a perfect human being! Is there any miracle greater than that? None that I know of. And if you are a parent, you'll attest to the fact that after the birth of your beautiful child, things begin to change quickly. Your child begins to grow and reach developmental milestones and eventually, even your grocery bills begin to go up! There is a lot of nurturing that happens, but beyond that you have no control over their automatic development and growth pattern. So 18 years later your child has gone from one cell to 95 trillion cells. Think of how many pairs of shoes you had to buy, and how big their hands got, what color their hair is, what color their eyes are-you had no control over that. That power is already in there. So as we sit here as adults, 180 billion of those 95 trillion cells will require repair or replacement today. How would you like to use your educated mind to deal with that? In addition, your heart is beating, your lungs are breathing, your food is digesting, and all your daily interactions are occurring. Amazing, isn't it?

# Chapter 3: It Starts with your Spine

*"Look well to the spine for the cause of disease."*
*- Hippocrates, Father of Medicine.*

So right now you're wondering how does this have anything to do with chiropractic and health care? Well, it's got everything to do with it because the way that innate power expresses itself in your body is through the nervous system. You have a brain and spinal cord, from which thirty-three pairs of nerves exit between your spinal joints. Those nerves transmit signals to every single organ, tissue and cell in your body. When I stated earlier that our bodies are designed to heal themselves, it's true, but that only works if your nervous system and its communication throughout the entire body is working perfectly. If it is, then your body is working, healing, and functioning the way it's supposed to.

# NEUROSURGEONS KNOW THE SECRET

One thing that researchers, chiropractors and physicians understand is that in order for the nerve system to work properly the way it was designed, the spine needs to be perfectly aligned. People often see neurosurgeons for radiating pain, neuralgia, and sciatica. Dr. Alf Breig, a Swedish neurosurgeon and Nobel Prize recipient, did some really interesting research on this. Dr. Breig studied patients coming in with cervical radiculopathy, which is radiating pain away from the site of origin, in this case was the neck. Common symptoms of this condition would be pain, numbness and tingling down the arms into the hands.

He took cervical x-rays of these people and he found that their spines were totally out of whack: they were either straight, the discs were worn out, or if they had a neck curve, it was going the wrong way. He hypothesized that if he recreated the natural curve in the neck it would take pressure off of the spinal cord, thus improving spinal cord function and restoring nerve transmission to the areas in the body experiencing radicular symptoms.

For his research, he operated on 200 people. He inserted wires on the back tips of each cervical (neck) vertebra by drilling a hole. He then weaved wires through and then cinched it up. It could be described as putting braces on one's neck. Essentially, he took the cervical spine from being straight and recreated a normal curve in it instantaneously. For the majority of the people, when they woke up from surgery, guess what happened to their symptoms? They were completely gone. They thought he was a miracle worker until they realized that they couldn't move their neck because of the wires! Although they didn't have any more radiating nerve pain, they had a blind spot the size of a barn. [13]

The conclusion was from this discovery is that if we can recreate the natural curve in the spine, we can alleviate a lot of health problems.

So if there could be a way that we could do that- without surgery, without drugs, without jeopardizing your long-term range of movement--would that be a good thing? Yes, and that is what today's corrective chiropractic is all about. It is about taking you from wherever you are and bringing you into normal proper alignment, removing nerve pressure and allowing the body to heal better. In the last decade, corrective chiropractic has also found that as the spine is re-aligned even the discs themselves will start to rehydrate and be restored. The body has a tremendous ability to heal itself.

## ALIGN THE SPINE AND YOU'LL BE FINE (MORE THAN FINE)

What does proper alignment of the spine look like? Your spine needs to be perfectly straight from the front and back, and needs 3 flowing curves when you look at it from the side. When that alignment and structural integrity is present, there's little to no wear and tear in the spine, and there's little to no stress on the nerve system. In this ideal position the spinal cord is relaxed inside the spine, and signals going from the spinal cord that allow for function, healing and recreation are able to happen optimally. Your body is in essence, working the way it was designed to work to its fullest potential.

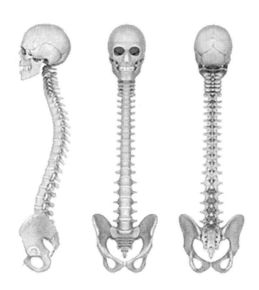

## STRESSORS CAUSE DIS-EASE

If we are designed to be well and our natural state is to be healthy then why do we get sick? Simply put, it is because of stress. As we spend more time on this earth we are exposed to many stresses.

The main life stressors that we experience can be divided into 3 categories. They are physical, chemical, and emotional. Most people think about physical stress first such as car accidents, sports injuries, poor work or sleeping habits. Did you know that for some of us, the first real physical stress we experienced in life was being born? .[14] Presently, with the increased use of computers, tablets, and cell phones combined with a sedentary lifestyle and poor posture habits at work and at rest, chiropractors are seeing more and more people developing what is commonly called "Text Neck", or "Computer Neck". [15]

Chemical stressors include things that are toxic to our bodies such as drugs, alcohol, smoking, medications, pesticides, unclean water and air.

Emotional stress can be anything from having a flat tire to grieving over a loved one. Your body's physiology will change instantly just from receiving bad news from a person who is a thousand miles away.

It doesn't matter what type of stress you have or go through, the body will always have one response for all three stressors. It is called the fight or flight response. In this response, your body goes through a number of quick changes to help you adapt to the sudden stress impending. Your pupils will dilate, you breathe quicker, your bowel movements slow down or stop altogether. Your immune system shuts off. Your stress hormone called cortisol will increase. Your heart beats faster. Your body will stop the blood flow to your hands and feet to save it for your heart resulting in that your hands and feet get cold. Your stomach produces acid; your muscles become your tense. This is all initially a normal sequence of responses so protect your most important organs in your body: your brain and your heart. And after a short period of stress— your body is designed to come out of its stress response and back to ease. This is a natural, innate adaption. However, if we continue to experience a  stressful event for a long duration of time, then this is when we run into trouble.

Everyone on the planet has the same posture response to stress and that is a flexed position. Think of a cat. If a cat gets stressed, what kind of posture does it assume? When we get stressed, we go into a flexed position, meaning our head goes forward and body curls down. And this is the chiropractic link: the spine and spinal cord is inside our body and goes into a flexed position too. If you stay in this flexed position over a long period of time, then the spine begins to wear out faster than it should. Let's take the neck for example.

If the head is forward, gravity is working through these

joints and these joints are going to wear out very quickly.[1617] That leads to degenerative disc disease, degenerative joint disease and arthritis of the spine. Many of our patients already know that they have arthritis - which causes a tremendous amount of pain and suffering.

But all of this pales by comparison to what is happening to the spinal cord when the head is flexed forward. As mentioned earlier, the neurosurgeon Dr. Alf Breig has shown that when the head is flexed forward the spinal cord stretches anywhere from 5 to 7 centimeters. They call that a tensile stretch or a tethering stress because the spinal cord is attached at the top of your skull and the bottom of your tailbone. In essence, it is stretching the spinal cord and is affecting the signals from the brain to the rest of the body.[18] And when you change forces, or put pressure on neural tissue, particularly the spinal cord, it changes the rate at which it fires the nerve signals. Essentially, it distorts the message system to the vital organs, arms and legs. For example, have you ever hit your 'funny bone'? That weird feeling you experience when that exposed nerve on your elbow gets hit, is exactly the same type of distortion that happens inside your spinal cord. The signal becomes distorted much like when you get fuzzy sound from when the dial on the radio is just a little bit off. If it isn't *exactly*, 106.5FM, you get a fuzzy sound and can't hear the message correctly. So in your body, if you distort the neural tissue coming out of the neck or out of the mid back and it is going to the heart, or lungs, or the kidney or the organs, it's going to distort it.

When you have distorted nerve signals or 'fuzziness' occurring for months, years or decades, the result will eventually lead to disease in the body. The signals become compromised to the point where your body can no longer adapt with a healthy response. A study was done where they looked at cadavers who had died from various diseases, like diseases of the heart, lung, kidney, colon. It was found that when they traced back the nerves that supplied the diseased organ to the place where they originated from the spine, there was a misalignment in the spine that had been compromising the nerve. That pressure on the nerve over a long period of time reduces nerve function and can thus affect its corresponding organ.[19]

Now just imagine going through life only hearing that fuzzy message. How hard does everything else become? If the body is not getting the clear nerve supply, there is no possible way for the body to function, heal or adapt properly And over time...living in 'fuzz', you will get tired, start giving up, and thinking to yourself that "This is as good as it gets", and just like our friend, Anne (remember her from the beginning?), you wake up one day, wondering what happened?

## KEEP YOUR HEAD ON STRAIGHT

Normal and healthy posture is essential for good health. Since we live in a forward facing world, the repetitive use of computers, TV, video games, trauma and even backpacks have forced the body to adapt to a forward head posture.

This result will cause neck and skull misplacement, leading to what is called "Forward Head Syndrome". In other words, your chin is out in front of your shoulders and chest. This leads to pathological tension on the spinal cord and brain stem.

# Here are some of the long-term consequences of Forward Head Syndrome:

1. Leads to long-term muscle strain, disc herniations and pinched nerves.[21]

2. Decreases respiratory muscle strength and function.[22] [23]

3. For every inch that the head is forward beyond normal results in an increase in the weight of the head on the spine by an additional 10 pounds.[24]

4. A loss of cervical curve stretches the spinal cord by 5-7cm and causes disease.[25]

5. 90% of stimulation and nutrition to the brain is generated by movement of the spine. Forward head posture adversely affects proper nutrition to the brain.[26]

6. Forward head posture can add up to 30 pounds of abnormal leverage pulling the entire spine out of alignment and may result in the loss of 30% of vital lung capacity.[27]

7. Loss of good bowel peristaltic function and evacuation is a common effect of Forward head posture.[28]

# Chapter 4: The Good News

Of course, there is good news! If a chiropractor finds your spine out of proper alignment, we get to fix it and restore it back to normal![29] And that is exactly what chiropractors do. We take the pressure off the spinal cord and nerve system, and help to remove the interference along the nerve system pathways. This allows the body to function and adapt properly— essentially fulfilling your body's natural ability to heal itself. This is good news because throughout this process you start experiencing your body's strong healing capabilities. Your body starts to function again. You go from dis-ease to ease. You start realizing just how amazing you truly are. You begin to experience health like you never would have ever imagined possible.

Let me share a story with you. I can tell you dozens of these stories, but this one is probably one of the most dramatic, and I'm telling you a dramatic story so you really get a good visual... but the power that healed this little girl that I'm going to tell you about is the same power that's in you and me. It's the same power that we help release with every single chiropractic adjustment. No matter what your problem is, whether it's a little bit of a neck pain, whether it's cancer, or heart disease or anything else.

Here's what happened: A woman started care with us and

about 2 weeks into her care, she said, "I have an 9-year-old daughter, and she is very ill. The doctors don't even know why she is always sick. She has had migraines 5 days a week and has been missing weeks of school." She went on to say, "We've seen all the specialists and no one knows what to do. I don't want to keep giving her drugs for the rest of her life. Is there anything you can do?" And our response was, "We have no idea if we can help, but bring her in for a chiropractic check-up, and if we find she has pressure on her nerve system, there may be something we can do."

So her mom brought Katlyn who is 9 years old and in such terrible pain in her head that she doesn't smile or say anything. Her history was at birth she had birth trauma via vacuum extraction, an APGAR score of 7. During the first few weeks of her life, she had difficulty breathing and by 5 months had an ear infection. Over the last 6 years of Katlyn's life, she has been on 15 rounds of antibiotics, and takes puffers for asthma from being diagnosed at age 2, and regularly takes Tylenol to help cope with her migraines.

We analyzed her spine and found that she had a spinal misalignment in her upper neck, which affects the nerves that supply the head. In addition, postural assessment showed her neck bending to the right and X- rays reveals a loss of normal neck curvature in her spine.

It was clear that Katlyn was getting less nerve supply to her body. In addition, she had a weakened immune system from an accumulation of toxins from antibiotics.

So we began to adjust this little girl with the goal to take the pressure off her nerve system, and allow the body to heal the way it was designed to. Initially, we adjusted her every day, and then 3x/week, and eventually we were able to take the pressure off and this little girl started to respond, because the signals to her brain were finally getting through to the rest of her body. Within the first month, her Mom noticed that she was not complaining of headaches. After 3 months, her Mom reported that she hasn't had to use her puffers anymore. After 6 months of chiropractic corrective care, there were remarkable changes on her x-ray showing a fully resorted healthy curve in her neck.

Now, Katlyn is able to function normally, and has never missed a day of school. She is a happy and healthy tween and has never taken a medication since she started chiropractic care.

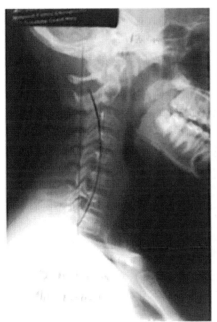 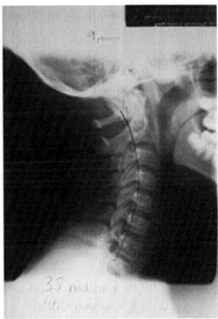

The story I've just reiterated is not to impress you, but to impress upon you that it wasn't us, it was the power that was already in there, from "above-down-inside-out."

That is the same power that is released every time a chiropractor performs a chiropractic adjustment and removes interference on your spinal cord, enabling your body to communicate and restore fully.

## YOU GET TO BE HEALTHY EVERY TIME

It is a shared opinion that every single time you are getting adjusted your body is getting healthier and healthier, regardless of symptoms. Why? Because every adjustment removes nerve interference and improves the connection between your brain and the body. Your brain/body connection is essential for everyday life functions including repair functions. For example, did you know that you get a brand new liver approximately every year? Approximately every 4 months all your red blood cells are wiped out and your body creates a completely new set. Your skin is replaced every month.

Your taste buds are replaced every 11 days, and your stomach lining is replaced every 5 days.[30] In order for this effective repair and replacement of tissues to occur, your brain and body need to be in constant communication.

When there is interference along the brain/body communication, your body cannot optimally do what it is designed to do. [31] However, with every single chiropractic adjustment, the goal is to remove that interference and thus enhance a better brain/body connection. The result is a better opportunity for your body to improve its capacity to heal, adapt and repair.[32]

Imagine what you could do, how much energy you could have, how productive and clear-minded you could be, if you used chiropractic as an approach to naturally enhancing your health and wellbeing.

# PART TWO:

## Your Guide to Abundant Health

# PUT ON YOUR OWN OXYGEN MASK FIRST

This is the safety instruction message given to all grown ups before a plane takes off. The same message applies to your health – you need to put your oxygen mask on first or you won't be good to anyone.

You have been given a body and a purpose to walk through your life with here on earth. In order to experience abundant health, you need to take care of yourself. However, the message of the mainstream mechanistic model is telling us the opposite. It says that you don't have to do anything to take care of your body because at the end of the road there is going to be a little pill or 'procedure' that is going to save your life and extend your life, and maybe give you a better quality of life. Yet that model hasn't come even close to fulfilling its promises.

As the old saying goes: "If you look after your body, your body will look after you." What are the things you need to do to be a good steward of your body?

You need to:

- Maintain an ideal body weight
- Eat well
- Exercise regularly
- Think positive thoughts
- Avoid drinking too much
- Never smoke
- Manage your stress—(and give yourself recovery time if you have stress)
- Limit TV time
- And of course, get adjusted!

Would you agree that if you do those simple things it would lead to a life of health and vitality? Now imagine doing the opposite of everything on that list. Let's say you're overweight, you're not eating well, you're not exercising, you're drinking too much, you're smoking, you have high stress and you are not dealing with it very well, you're sitting in front of the TV all day, and there is a disconnect between your brain and your body. How do you think you are going to function? Obviously not well. That kind of lifestyle leads to disease, and destruction, and early death. You may have been ordained to live for 100 years, but if you don't look after yourself, the chances of you making it are not very good.

In the following chapters, you will find the 8 essential lifestyle steps that you can do right now to improve your health and well-being, and live the life you were called to live.

# Chapter 5: Get Adjusted for the Health of it!

## FIND A CHIROPRACTOR WHO DOES CORRECTIVE CARE

My husband and I have been in practice since 1999. When we first started out, we used to do what is called 'patch it' chiropractic where you give a patient a few adjustments and help to get them out of pain and then send them on their way. We did that because that is what we learned in chiropractic school. The problem was that we were finding so many patients came back to see us a few months later with the same problems, and sometimes it would even get worse! We were so frustrated because we couldn't understand why the same problems kept coming up and they were not getting better. Out of that frustration, we began to explore other Chiropractic techniques and procedures so that we could truly help improve our patients' health. What we discovered is called corrective chiropractic care where we could restore the spine to back to its ideal alignment.[33]

The more we started focusing on correcting the spine and restoring it to its normal state, the more incredible health transformations we saw in our patients because their bodies were truly healing at a greater capacity. Our goal was to restore the spine back to normal alignment, reduce spinal cord stress, and thus improve communication along their neural pathways. As a result, patients not only experienced resolution from neck and or back pain, but their asthma, digestion, sleep problems, ear infections and other ailments would improve and even resolve. We even have diabetic patients who have experienced improved insulin levels to the point of being able to decrease their insulin intake because their body was able to properly adapt again. Patients with high blood pressure began to experience normal blood pressure again. Heartburn, digestive issues, and even eyesight was reported to have improved. We began seeing the changes on x-rays as well. As their spinal alignment improved there would be noticeable evidence of reversed arthritis along the spine. [34] We, along with hundreds of other chiropractors, continue to train and practice corrective chiropractic care in conjunction with promoting a healthy lifestyle to patients. As a result, thousands of patients across the world continue to experience massive health transformations that truly last a lifetime.

Note: In the "Frequently Asked Questions" section of this book, you will find all the answers to your questions about health and chiropractic in more detail.

# Corrective chiropractic care

is designed to help restore the proper position of spinal bones much like dental braces are used to rehab crooked tooth.

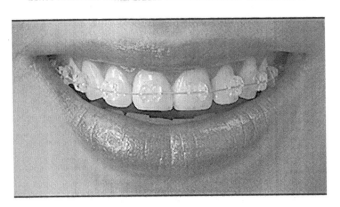

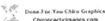

Done For You Chiro Graphics
ChiropracticImages.com

By now, you might be wondering how is this possible? Or why haven't I heard about this before? Well, chiropractic care doesn't have an annual billion dollar advertising budget like the pharmaceutical companies do. The truth is, at this stage, chiropractors simply can't spend billions of dollars to let the world know the truth of where your health comes from. One day we will. So instead of being exposed to powerful messages about the benefits of chiropractic care, the general population is bombarded with messages from commercials and advertisements about a pill for every ill. Most people find out about corrective chiropractic care from word of mouth, local and global outreach, social media, or discovering it by reading a book like this.

## IS CHIROPRACTIC GLAMOROUS?

Chiropractic might not be as appealing as showing off your fit and toned body at the gym, or putting up a beautiful photo of the nutritious food you made on Instagram. Not everyone gets so excited about pre and post x-rays that they post it on Facebook. But Chiropractic is based on the timeless truth that health comes from 'above down inside out.' It is the cornerstone for every other lifestyle habit in order to truly thrive. It turns your power on! The healing power inside you is like Love; you can't describe it truly until you experience it. It is the reason why people who get chiropractic adjustments are smiling because it is a reflection of what is manifesting within. It's the main ingredient and when you add all the other great lifestyle practices to it—you experience an abundant life. This is the life you are destined for!

> *"Two roads diverged in a wood and I --*
> *I took the one less traveled by,*
> *And that has made all the difference."*
> *-Robert Frost*

## IMPORTANT NOTE FOR THE REST OF PART 2:

I'm a Chiropractor, and like all chiropractors, we are experts at adjusting people's spines. That's our gift! We don't do massage, even though Chiropractors are trained and can give a decent massage. We are just not massage therapists so we would rather refer out to someone who is an expert at massage. The same principle applies to many aspects of this section as well. I can give you the "Coles Notes" on what I know professionally so that you can take your health to a higher level immediately. However, I do suggest that you seek out the distinct professional for further specific concerns. For example, consult a personal trainer to further your fitness levels, or a homeopath to help with addressing specific ailments, or read "It Starts With

Food" by Dallas and Melissa Hartwig, "Grain Brain" by David Perlmutter, or "The Bulletproof Diet" by Dave Asprey, to clean up your diet.

# Chapter 6: Get Moving!

Did you know that 90% of the stimulation and nutrition to the brain is generated by the movement of the spine? Just like whole food is nutrition for your body, movement is nutrition for your brain and health.[35] When you move, receptors in your spine send signals to your brain to improve your immune system. All research that studies preventing heart disease, improving brain function, reducing stress and promoting weight loss, point to regular exercise. This is a no-brainer.

Did you know that sitting is the new smoking and sitting has actually joined smoking and obesity as an important risk factor for chronic disease and premature death?[36]

According to a study in the British Medical Journal, just by reducing average sitting time to less than 3 hours per day could increase your life expectancy by 2 years.[37] In fact, people who sat for the longest periods of time were twice as likely to have diabetes or heart disease, compared to those who sat the least.[38]

The more you sit, the less your body wants to move, so if you find yourself in a place where you are sitting for long periods of time, make it so that either you are active sitting (on a gym ball) or set a timer so that you are not sitting for long periods. Your body will thank you.

If you find yourself in a place where you feel stuck, do

yourself a favor and sign up for an exercise class. There you will have direction and accountability and momentum. As a bonus, you will be immersed in a culture of people with similar desires to be fit and healthy. That is a great influence for creating sustainable change.

One of the biggest deterrents for people not signing up for an exercise class is the fact that they feel embarrassed by being the 'newbie' or intimidated by these so-called 'gym-people' who seem to be super fit, and have all the shiny tech gear. The truth is, everyone goes through this initially. The first class I ever went to was after my second pregnancy and I was quite out of shape. It was an aerobics class and I thought I was going to faint from feeling so out of place. Of course, what I didn't realize was that half the people in the class felt the same way! I got through that first class, and felt so good afterwards that I decided to go back again. Now I'm a regular. The point is, don't let your history dictate your destiny. Just take the next step and sign up.

## RUNNING, SWIMMING, SPINNING, PILATES, YOGA, AND INTERVAL TRAINING

When it comes to movement, what exercise is best? Anything that gets you excited inside and out. If you are passionate about biking, then biking you should do. Swimming is another great low impact exercise that you can get great results within a short period of time. Running is one of the most affordable exercises as you just need a pair of sneakers to get going.

If you have never jogged before and you would like to get started, sign up for a local "Learn to Run" class, or get a friend to join you for a set weekly jog. I personally enjoy Crossfit classes for its cross-training strategy and accountability.

If you are the disciplined type, then there are many great exercise programs on iTunes you can purchase and run off your computer or laptop to do at home on a regular basis. Jillian Michaels has a 30-minute strength cardio program with little to no equipment needed. The Daily Method DVD is a postural-based Pilates/yoga program and is fantastic for core stability and stretching. My personal all-time favorite app is called the 12minuteathleteworkout and is totally worth the $2.99 investment. You can find it on iTunes for loads of quality workouts that you can do in 12 minutes and no gym is needed.

When in doubt, just grab your sneakers and commit to just 20 minutes outside in the fresh air.

Lastly, if you really want to maximize your exercise with minimal time, try incorporating a Tabata style of exercise. It is a high-intensity interval training workout, known as HIIT, with rest periods that has shown to produce amazing fitness and health results alike. One study published in the *Journal of Obesity* reported that 12 weeks of high-intensity interval training not only can result in significant reductions in total abdominal, trunk, and visceral fat, but also can give you significant increases in fat-free mass and aerobic power.[39] Another study found that unfit but otherwise healthy middle-aged adults were able to improve their insulin sensitivity and blood sugar regulation after just two weeks of interval training (three sessions per week)[40]. As always when beginning a new fitness program, make sure to consult your family doctor.

Here is an excellent method that can be used whether you are running, biking, swimming, jumping, or dancing. If done correctly, you will experience great results:

- Warm up with a slow paced jog, bike or swim for 10 minutes.

- Exercise as hard and fast as you can for 30 seconds. You should be gasping for breath and feeling like you couldn't possibly go on another few seconds.

- Recover for 90 seconds, still moving, but at a slower pace and decreased resistance

- Repeat the high-intensity exercise and recovery 7 more times.

- Cool down for a few minutes afterward by cutting down your intensity by 50-80 percent[41]

If you need a timer for this type of interval training, you can either download a free "Tabata timer" app from iTunes, or set a sport watch to accommodate the interval times.

You can also check out the amazing people at HIITit.ca. For under a dollar, you will receive a live 12-minute workout right in your inbox every single day. No equipment needed and anyone can do it. Just 12 minutes! Visit drjodycox.com to get their promotional discount.


## RANGE OF MOTION IN 90 SECONDS

Range of Motion exercises will help you develop symmetry and coordination of movement that we continually lose through our repetitive asymmetrical work and lifestyle habits. The symmetry of movement will force the two halves of your brain to engage and integrate. Lack of proper and repeated integration of the brain has been shown to cause learning disabilities and difficulty with problem solving on a cognitive level (how you think) as well as an emotional level.

The Range of Motion exercises should take only 90 seconds to complete, and leave you feeling energized and alert. These exercises are not going to replace your chiropractic adjustment, but they are going to maximize the results of your adjustment and help you hold the adjustments longer. You can do them daily and at the beginning of your day as a way to 'lubricate' your joints; and also do them in the middle of your busy day, so you may break up the patterns of disconnectedness or idle tendencies.

## YOUR 90 SECONDS MOVEMENT DOWNLOAD

To download your copy of this amazing series of poses all formatted on one sheet that you can print out, visit my website at www.drjodycox.com.

# Chapter 7: Eat to Thrive

If you give the highest grade of gas to a broken down car, it really won't affect the performance of the car. It is better to first begin correcting the broken down car and then start giving it that great gas. I see so many people spending crazy amounts of money on organic food and supplements, but they don't take care of the spine and nervous system. It is your nervous system which controls everything in your body, including digestive function and cellular function. It's not the kale that cures cancer—it is the way your body utilizes the nutrients from the kale. It makes sense to invest in optimizing your nervous system so that when you consume all these great foods, you will have a better return on investment. Many times I see patients with poor posture who complain of poor digestion. There are two reasons behind this. One, if you are hunched over, structurally, there is less expansive space for your inner vital organs like your heart, lungs and stomach. When you have great posture, and you are not slouched, your organs are not cramped or crowded by structural constraints. The second issue is when your spine is excessively bent over in the mid back area, the excessive tensile spinal cord stress and pressure on exiting nerves in the spine cannot optimally supply those associated vital organs. The result could be anywhere from sluggish digestion to acid reflux.[42] [43] By correcting the spine and maintaining great posture, the function of the vital digestive organs can function optimally thus are able to maximize the nutritional value and energy supply from the food you enjoy.

Our food philosophy is this: We LOVE food. Every opportunity we get, we enjoy creating a nourishing whole food meal for our family that is attached to the vision we have for our lives. We can't stand labels. They force a person to define themselves with very rigid terms, and beat themselves up if they suddenly eat something that doesn't fit that definition. For that reason, we don't talk about trending diets like "the Paleo Diet" or the "Raw Food movement", etc.

"If something is new, it is probably not true. If it is true, it is probably not new." While it is important to stay current with research, be sure you make dietary adjustments based on timeless truths and line that up with what works best for your body. Finally, don't fall into the trap of idolizing some new food movement. Ultimately, it is more important what comes out of your mouth than what goes in your mouth.

Our family tries to eat mainly organic local food. We have a nice garden in our backyard and enjoy the harvest throughout the year. We shop at farmers' markets, we place orders for bulk frozen organic blueberries, and we will take advantage of some of the high-end quality products for reduced prices at Costco. Our diet has been consistently 50% plant-based, 25% meat (wild fish and sardines, grass fed organic beef, chicken, turkey and eggs), 15% quality fats (coconut oil, ghee, hemp hearts, and nuts), 5% whole organic grain (oats, quinoa, brown or wild rice), and 5% 'don't sweat the small stuff' foods. By that I mean organic wine and quality chocolate and sweets. We enjoy local eggs and wild fish at least two times a week, raw organic dairy or kefir regularly, and love our local honey. We drink loads of green and herbal teas as well. And yes, we love our coffee, too – black of course.

By eating this way, we *never* count calories or worry about our weight because we know that if we eat this way, our bodies will be in an excellent state of balance and health, naturally,

You don't have to give up *anything* you <u>really</u> love to be a healthier person, because I think that deprivation and/or eating with the feeling of guilt is far more detrimental to one's health than the food itself. Having said that, when you have a plan or vision for your life, the healthier choices become that much easier to make.

## SHUT DOWN AND SIT UP

We live in a world where multitasking has become a habit and is starting to influence our meals at the table. This distraction creates a disconnect between your meal and your mouth. Have you ever found yourself eating a meal while reading the paper or watching TV? Then you find yourself surprised when you look down at your plate to see that it is all gone. You don't even know what happened. You might even find yourself going back for more because you aren't even sure if you ate enough. Most likely, you didn't even chew your food enough for effective digestion. And while food is fuel for our bodies, it is not meant to be taken for granted.

Try shutting down all media and phones. Put the newspaper or book away and sit down (even for 15 minutes) to IN-JOY your meal. Allow no distraction from you actually connecting your nourishment to your body—so that you can actually enjoy the flavors and *feel* when you are completely satisfied. To re-appreciate your food again, try closing your eyes while chewing for a few bites. You will be surprised. Also, try smiling when you are eating--it will elevate all aspects of what a good whole meal is for—nurturing and nourishing your body and soul.

# EAT WHOLE FOOD FIRST

Yes, it sounds simple, and it really *is* simple. Eating whole foods means foods that have not been processed or are as close to their natural state as possible. For example, even if the label on the cheesy puffs bag says 'natural ingredients', is no longer in its natural form. All the ingredients had to been processed and then assembled before it could be packaged and consumed. A pear, on the other hand, is in its natural whole state, and is not processed. Whole foods contain the best building blocks that are essential for keeping you healthy.

Tip: You will save yourself a lot of time and money by shopping the perimeter of the grocery store. Once you decide to consume more whole foods, you will not be standing in an aisle comparing products or wasting time scrutinizing over a label trying to decide if it's 'slightly' healthy. Typically you find the majority of whole unprocessed foods around the perimeter of the grocery store. So take a lap, and enjoy the bounty.

# PLANT YOURSELF

A plant based diet means just that- a diet that is purely vegetables, fruits, nuts and seeds. The vast majority of people in North America do not consume nearly enough vegetables. [44] And if they do, it is mainly a few favorites: carrots, peas, tomatoes and potatoes. Almost every vegetable that has been studied has been found to contain substances that benefit the heart and blood or counteract the formation of tumors. Fresh vegetables, eaten with the right fats on a daily basis, are one of our best protections against coronary heart disease and cancer. The best source of dietary fiber comes from plants. Plant based foods with the highest sources of fiber are: berries, almonds, cauliflower, broccoli, Brussels sprouts, chia, flax, and root vegetables like sweet potatoes.[45]

Steaming is the best way to cook most vegetables as it preserves most vitamins, minerals and enzymes. While I do suggest incorporating raw vegetables, some vegetables are best eaten cooked. For example, raw cabbage, broccoli, Brussels sprouts and kale contain chemicals that block the production of the thyroid hormone (known medically as goitrogens). Raw beet greens, spinach and chard contain oxalic acid that blocks calcium and iron absorption and irritates the mouth and intestinal tract. Cooking these vegetables slightly destroys or neutralizes these harmful substances (as does the fermentation process). [46]

Make sure to try a variety of vegetables, and not just one type. The reason is if you eat something in excess, it can cause an adverse or allergic reaction. I typically aim for different 'rainbow' of vegetables and fruit, as each color of the plant contains different essential nutrients, but also because you get to experience a visual delight while you enjoy different flavors.

I attribute my clean living diet to one of the reasons why I have bounds of sustainable energy, sharp mental focus, excellent digestion, a vibrant complexion, and for the most part, an even emotional balance.

## GET FAT

What?!! Yes, you read that right. Get your fats right.

First things first: *Fat does not make you fat.*

In fact, it is just about the opposite. Good quality fat actually aids in metabolism and aids in the prevention of disease. Contrary to what has been preached to us over the past two decades, obesity has nothing to do with fat, but everything to do with overconsumption of carbohydrates. [47]

A study was done on people who limited carbohydrate intake but ate as much fat and protein as they wanted. They found that they lost more weight on average than those who avoided fats and increased carbohydrates, suggesting that fats don't make people fat. Excessive carbohydrates make people fat.

Here is how it works in a nutshell: Insulin is a hormone that is our body's primary regulator of sugar and fat metabolism. Insulin levels in the bloodstream are primarily determined by the amount of carbohydrates we consume. An excess of carbohydrates will break down into sugar and will result in an overwhelming surplus of insulin. The more insulin, the more we store fat. The less insulin, the more we can use fat for our body's energy needs.

Now that you know fat does not make you fat, you need to know the second fat fact:

*Fat is necessary for your health!*

Your brain is the fattest organ in the body and is made up of 60% fat.[48] Fat is an excellent source of energy and critical to supplying your organs, cells and hormones.

And the third thing is:

*Fat quality is important.*

Just because you now know that fat doesn't make you fat doesn't mean you can go ahead and eat anything containing fat in it. There are many different products with different types of fat, and also many deceiving sugars embedded along.

As you read the next section on sugars below, you will soon find out that fat and sugars play an interchangeable role in our health. If you do it right, you can experience tons of energy and improved weight metabolism and a prevention or great reduction of many diseases. If you do it wrong, however, you will be heading towards a perpetual health disaster! So get this part straight.

There are different types of fats, but for simplicity, consider there are two types of fats: Bad Fats and Good Fats.

The bad fats are vegetable oils, canola oil, seed oils (sunflower), and transfats. Often you will see these on labels as 'partially hydrogenated' in packaged foods. Transfats are the worst and can contribute to heart disease. But you don't have to worry about this too much now, if you start eating whole foods and reducing your processed foods, right?!

Good fats come from pastured grass-fed animals, wild fish, eggs, butter, ghee, extra virgin olive oil, olives, nuts, avocados, and coconut.

Don't be afraid of saturated fats when they are sourced from pastured grass fed animals. It is not the saturated content in meat that causes heart disease as we had been led to believe. It is the toxic contaminants in the factory-farming system that contributes to the problem. Residues from antibiotics and injected hormones are stored in the fat of the animal. When we consume the fat from these animals, we are also ingesting these toxins.[49] It is the accumulation of these toxins which are contributing to many health-related diseases.

On the other hand, when you consume grass fed meats, they are high in Omega 3s which are your anti-inflammatory essential fats. They reduce blood clotting, blood pressure, allergy response, water and sodium retention by the kidneys, while also increasing immunity. Omega 3s reduce the risk of cardiovascular events, diabetes, and modulate gene expression.

Omega 6 on the other hand, if consumed in too high amounts can do quite the opposite.[50] Conventional grain fed meats have much higher doses of Omega 6 essential fatty acids and should not be consumed.

## WATCH YOUR SUGARS, YOU ARE SWEET ENOUGH

Did you know that refined sugar is a toxic substance that is more addictive than cocaine? This includes high fructose corn syrup, and processed sugar, which is found in fruit juice, pop, and packaged foods (read your labels).[51]

Here is the deal on sugar. It is everywhere and I bet if you did a three-day inventory of your diet, you would find it in surprising places: breads, crackers, pasta, fruit, dairy, and meat (yes even many deli meats have sugar in them). Not to mention the obvious: cookies, candy bars and even seemingly healthy juices (even those organic juices you think are healthy are loaded with sugar!).

Sugar can best be compared to rocket fuel – your body needs it for quick powerful boosts - while fat, the body's preferred source for everything else, is like diesel fuel; it burns longer and stronger. The purpose of glucose in the body is to feed the brain and to be converted to glycogen for easy and quick access in the muscles and liver. However, when consuming highly processed foods or refined sugars in large quantities, that extra sugar cannot be utilized in our body and ends up overwhelming our organs. This causes all kinds of inflammatory conditions such as diabetes, metabolic dysfunction and brain disease—not to mention an increase in our waistlines.

It's not that a treat once in a while isn't OK. It the over-consumption of grain-based carbohydrates that is causing toxic overload. Breads, pastas, muffins, pizza, french fries, corn and rice are very high in carbohydrates. These carbohydrate laden foods are broken down by our digestive system into sugar and then stored as fat, which lingers and overwhelms our bodies.

Not only that but because of its addictive properties, the more sugar you consume, the more you crave. It is not easy to eliminate sugar, and it may seem impossible at first, but once you make the changes, you will start experiencing immediate changes in your body and health.

## POSITIVELY PROTEIN

Protein is essential for life. It is required for growth and development of bones, muscles, nerves, the brain, skin, hair, nails, tendons and ligaments. Your hormones are part protein. Your enzymes are proteins. Your neurotransmitters are proteins. The antibodies of your immune system are proteins. DNA, your genetic material, is a code for building proteins. Every single cell in the body needs protein.

Back when I was a vegetarian, I witnessed many people who claimed to be vegetarian, but didn't get adequate sources of protein, nor did they consume ample amount of vegetables. They were just supplementing their meat avoidance with breads and pastas, which again was excessive in refined carbohydrates. All plants have protein so it is important that if you are vegetarian to make sure you are eating enough vegetables to fill your daily requirement. Plants abundant in protein are dark leafy vegetables, alfalfa sprouts and spirulina.

Ultimately, it comes down to how nutritious a diet is overall and how well the nutrients are absorbed by the body. For example, a 6 oz. Steak has 40g of protein, but when you cook it, only 20g is usable by the body. Even then, the body needs to break down the protein in the meat into amino acids so it can be absorbed. This takes a lot of energy by the body.

When you eat raw fruits and vegetables, the protein is already in amino acid form, and is much easier to absorb and be utilized by the body. Looking at it from a calorie perspective, 100 calories of ground beef has 10 grams of protein while 100 calories of fresh baby spinach has 12 grams of protein. Calorie per calorie, spinach has more protein than beef. That being said, a bed of spinach salad will not fill you up in any way so make sure you are getting another source of nutrient dense protein.

Great sources of nutrient dense protein are grass fed organic meat, sustainable seafood, whole eggs, full fat organic dairy or kefir, nuts or organic tempeh. In my opinion, it is of vital importance that you have good quality meat. Conventional meat has unfavorable fatty acid ratio; higher levels of the inflammatory omega 6 fats and lower levels of the anti-inflammatory omega 3 fats (the good fats). It is the conventional meat (particularly the fatty areas) that has the added hormones, antibiotics, herbicides and GMOs (Genetically Modified Organisms) in it that get passed onto you. (Refer back to the 'Get Fat' section above)

By the way, you will offset the costs of buying good quality meat by reducing your packaged processed food purchases.

As I mentioned before, as much as I love and know about the value of good nutrition, my true expertise is Chiropractic. For further exploration and a detailed explanation on eating for good health, I recommend reading "It Starts With Food" by Dallas and Melissa Hartwig, and also "Grain Brain" by David Perlmutter, or "The Bulletproof Diet" by Dave Asprey.

# SUPPLEMENTS

Many people feel like they are not getting enough nutrients from the foods they consume these days, and need to supplement by taking vitamins. Before buying a whole bunch of supplements, review your diet first to see if it needs some adjusting to get the properly balanced nutrients. All too often I see people consume copious amounts of vitamins, spending tons of money, while their daily diet is loaded with poor animal fats (meaning not grass fed, organic), sugars, dairy, and processed foods. Once you have a well-developed diet, full of lots of plant based foods, good quality animal protein, healthy fats and water, then the next step is to supplement in areas where some extra nutritional boosting is necessary to create an optimal environment.

The fabulous four supplements I recommend to fulfill what is missing for the majority of people are this simple formula: ABCDs and big Mama M!

**Acidophilus**: Probiotics are strains of healthy bacteria known to help digest food and strengthen our immune system. Your body is made up of around ten trillion cells, but you harbor *a hundred* trillion bacteria.[52] The problem is that we kill off many of the good essential bacteria from poor nutrition, medications and stressful lifestyles. The goal is to help keep the good bacteria plentiful in your body. Taking a probiotic can help ensure this. Be sure to rotate your probiotics around. If you take the same probiotic every time, you are only addressing a small spectrum of bacteria. If you mix it in your diet by rotating probiotics found in kefir, and fermented products like sauerkraut and kombucha, as well as take good quality probiotics supplement, then you will be able to address broader spectrums of the bacteria ecology within your body.

**B-Complex Vitamin** The Vitamin B family is a useful group that targets some of the most common health issues of modern society, including fatigue, stress, depression, high cholesterol and brain and heart health.

**Cod Liver Oil or Quality Fish Oil 2-4g/day:** Essential Fatty acids are critical structural components for cellular function and the body's physiological function. Because we eat grains and vegetable oils, and because we eat domesticated grain-fed animals, we consume way too much omega-6 fats, which lead to inflammation. The ratio of omega-3 to omega-6 in most people is so imbalanced it causes people to be unhealthy and can contribute to many diseases from heart disease to ADHD. [53]

Balancing with high quality Omega-3 fish oil has proven to decrease inflammation in the body and promotes good heart and joint health. It has also been shown to be a natural antidepressant,[54] which, along with exercise, beats any medication out there. Deficiency in omega 3 fatty acids impairs memory and brain function, worse than the effects of sugar.[55]

**Vitamin D 4000-8000/day for Adults[56]** Vitamin D is a fat-soluble vitamin that we obtain mainly from sunlight. It plays an important role in our overall health, including keeping your bones and teeth strong. It is also important for modulating the immune system, and reducing the risk of diabetes (type 1 and type 2). In fact, supplementing with vitamin D3 has the potential to reduce cancer deaths by 75%. [57]

The majority of naturally obtained vitamin D is synthesized on the skin when a form of cholesterol comes in contact with UV rays from the sun. The ideal way to get it is from sun exposure (without sunscreen). In Canada, we have less exposure to sunshine given our latitude on the map, and therefore, it is essential that we supplement during the fall, winter and spring months.

**Magnesium:** Magnesium is known as the calming supplement. It helps to relax muscles and is known to aid in a good night's sleep. It is fundamental in keeping your heart rhythm steady and bones strong. Many studies point out that environmental stress, emotional stress, and physical stress will contribute to a decrease in the body's natural magnesium content. I recommend the brand Natural Calm and we sip it in hot water as a night warming tea before bedtime.

## KEEP THE WATER RUNNING

It is so important to drink pure water on a regular basis. I am not talking about juices, coffee or tea. In fact, many people say they are getting enough water through these beverages, but in fact, it creates the opposite effect on the body. It is true these beverages contain water, but they also contain dehydrating agents as well and therefore end up causing dehydration.

The color of your urine will help you determine whether or not you might need to drink more. As long as you are not taking Vitamin B2 (found in most multi- vitamins) which turns your urine bright yellow, then your urine should be very light-colored yellow. If it is deep, dark yellow then you are likely not drinking enough water.

As we age, the water content in your cells decreases, and as a result decreases cellular function and volume, making your cells sluggish or inefficient. [58] Drinking water on a regular daily basis is vital for not only proper cell function, but it hydrates your muscles, helps to flush out your digestive system and helps to restore and maintain energy levels. Just think how tired you are when you are dehydrated. A dry mouth is the last sign of dehydration. I hear many people tell me that they keep forgetting to drink water, so here is a simple plan I use to help get you started on rehydrating your body.

First thing in the morning upon waking: warm water with a squeeze or two of fresh lemon.

Then: 10am water 2pm water 4pm water

TIP: buy a BPA-free water container with a straw. I have the ones from Starbucks, but you can find them anywhere. When you have a glass of water with a straw, you are more likely to drink it all (than sip it periodically).

## SUPER FOODS

The way we define super foods is they are foods that are super concentrated and highly nutritious, and function to promote health or prevent disease. Consider them like a spice that you can add to your already amazing foods to enhance your nutrition in a meal or rebalance a neglected healthy diet.

**Hemp hearts**: These are seeds of the plant Cannabis sativa, and they provide a broad spectrum of health benefits including: weight loss, increased and sustained energy, rapid recovery from disease or injury, lowered cholesterol and blood pressure, reduced inflammation, improvement in circulation and immune system as well as natural blood sugar control. Hemp hearts contain a perfect balance of protein, (about 30%), essential fats, vitamins and enzymes. 8 Tbsp. of hemp hearts provides 1.75 times more protein than a litre of mother's milk.

**Chia**: These are tiny little black seeds that contain more beneficial omega 3 fats than a piece of salmon and 3 to 6 times more calcium than a glass of milk. Just 1 tablespoon of Chia contains 11 grams of good fiber which is nearly 50% of the daily recommended dose that helps to prevent colon disorders like diverticulitis or IBS. As for protein, it is considered a complete protein as it contains essential amino acids which when synthesized, build strong healthy tissues.

We use chia in our granola or soak it overnight in almond milk and add to porridge.

**Cacao**: Cacao is not cocoa. They may look very similar, smell the same, feel the same, they are even spelled almost the same way, but they are worlds apart when it comes to nutrition. Cacao is the raw form of chocolate while cocoa is the heated form. It is theorized by Raw foodies that when you heat any food over 104°F, you destroy enzymes and vitamins that are in it and as a result, the once nutrient dense food now becomes only just a tasty one. That is not to say that cooked food isn't good for you because it definitely has its place in the diet, but raw chocolate versus a Hershey bar? There's simply no comparison. Cacao has multiple health benefits including antioxidants and magnesium. The essential fatty acids found in chocolate may help the body to raise good cholesterol and lower bad cholesterol. In addition, it also contains the 'bliss' nutrient called Theobromine, which gives you that pleasant sensation. Now, don't go into devouring Cacao to be happy. But it is theorized to help boost your happy state. And hey, let's face it—who isn't happy enjoying chocolate? We add Cacao nibs in a nut mix that I make, or you can blend it with a frozen banana to make a nice chocolate ice-cream dessert.

**Spirulina**: One of the great super foods. It's approximately 65 to 71 percent complete protein in its natural state, higher than virtually any other unprocessed food. And unlike most other forms of protein, the protein in spirulina is 85-95% digestible. This is a great way to maintain a high quality of absorbable protein in your diet, especially if you are vegan (no meat, nor dairy). Spirulina contains a lot of an omega 6 called gamma linolenic acid (GLA).[59]

The amount is second only to that in mother's milk. GLA is anti-inflammatory and good for allergies. You can buy spirulina in a powder form and add it to water or coconut water for a refreshing drink.

**Coconut Oil**: Is one of those amazing foods that can be universally used in almost everything from skin care to baking. We use it in lieu of nasty margarine and it has incredible health benefits. This includes stimulating your metabolism and giving you more energy. Coconut oil has the ability to be antiviral, anti-fungus and antibacterial. Placed on the skin, coconut oil does wonders for any eczema, infections and even fungus of the nails. Taken internally it has been known to keep the colon healthy, inhibits yeast and candida growth and feeds the body with instant energy. Coconut Oil has one important asset: it contains Lauric Acid, which in the body has strong immune boosting effects. (Another high source of Lauric Acid is mother's milk.) I am referring to extra virgin organic coconut oil as compared to hydrogenated coconut oil -- which incidentally was how coconut oil came to earn its bad reputation in the first place because the research was done on the inferior hydrogenated (processed) oil.

**Turmeric**: The yellow spice is long known for its anti-inflammatory and antioxidant properties. It is known to aid in easing acute arthritic pain, boosting circulation, and soothing the digestive tract. It also provides nourishment to your skin and helps prevent wrinkles. Now who wouldn't want that?

**Quinoa**: Quinoa (pronounced keen-wah) is considered to be a "whole grain" but it is actually the seed of a plant that is a relative of leafy green vegetables like spinach and Swiss chard. It is an energy-rich food that delivers heaps of fiber and protein but very little fat and no gluten. The protein quinoa is a complete protein, meaning that it includes all nine essential amino acids. Quinoa's amino acid profile is well balanced, making it a good choice for vegans concerned about adequate protein intake. And because quinoa is a very good source of manganese as well as a good source of magnesium, iron, copper and phosphorous, this grain may be especially valuable for persons with migraine headaches, diabetes and atherosclerosis.

**Green tea**: My favorite daytime drink has cardiovascular and cancer preventative characteristics due to its antioxidant properties. It is used in the treatment of arthritic disease as an anti-inflammatory. The antioxidant in green tea is 100 times more effective than vitamin C and 24 times better than vitamin E. It also helps to burn fat and boosts your metabolism naturally.

## A WORD ON "ORGANIC"

Pesticide residues have been found on 65 percent of food even *after* they had been washed or peeled.[60] Pesticides damage your nervous system, affect your hormones and can cause cancer.[61] [62] We all know organic choices are the best choices, but it can add up. We always buy grass fed meat, which can be expensive; however, we don't consume very much packaged or processed foods (which are very expensive). so it offsets our budget and allows us to buy really good quality foods. That being said, even the organic choices in produce can be very expensive at times. I just can't justify spending $5 on one red pepper. So I will alter our weekly meal schedule until those organic red peppers are on sale or in season. In addition, you can rinse nonorganic vegetables in a sink full of water with ½ cup of apple cider vinegar to help remove some of the pesticides on your produce. To help save some money, follow the 'dirty dozen' system as researched by the Environmental Working Group (EWG), where you buy only organic for the top 12 foods that if bought conventionally, are the highest rated in pesticides:

| The Dirty Dozen (in order of contamination) | The Clean 15 (in order of least contamination) |
|---|---|
| Apples | Onions |
| Celery | Sweet Corn |
| Sweet bell peppers | Pineapples |
| Peaches | Avocado |
| Strawberries | Cabbage |
| Nectarines | Sweet Peas |
| Grapes | Asparagus |
| Spinach | Mangoes |
| Lettuce | Eggplant |
| Cucumbers | Kiwi |
| Blueberries | Cantaloupe |
| Potatoes | Sweet Potatoes |
|  | Grapefruit |
|  | Watermelon |
|  | Mushrooms |

## IN OUR HOME KITCHEN

Do you ever wonder what's in someone's kitchen cupboard? Many people are asking what do healthy Chiropractors eat? Well, if you walked into our kitchen today, here is what you would find:

## FOR YOUR PANTRY

- Organic Gluten Free oats
- Almond/spelt/coconut flour

- Homemade almond butter and hazelnut butter
- Brown rice pasta and quinoa pasta, and brown rice vermicelli
- Ascorbic Acid Powder
- Now Vitamin D & K2 capsules
- Natural Calm Magnesium powder
- Basmati rice, quinoa
- Extra virgin olive oil and Avocado Oil
- Balsamic vinegar
- Organic coconut sugar
- Local honey
- Organic maple syrup
- Medjool dates and dried figs
- Home dehydrated dried apricots, cherries, and mangoes
- Extra virgin coconut oil. This is a staple in our home – we use it for cooking, baking and for moisturizing our skin! It's an all-around amazing product.
- Bulletproof Brain Octane Oil-a concentrated pure coconut oil used for Bulletproof Coffee.
- Raw almonds - unsalted
- Raw pumpkin seeds, macadamia nuts, sunflower seeds, cashews, hazelnuts, walnuts, pecans, coconut flakes (we reserve a drawer for these)
- Salt & pepper grinders - organic Celtic or Himalayan sea salt only!
- ANY spice. A really good spice rack is a great investment. Cinnamon is great for

adding sweetness to oatmeal or just on chopped apples/pears. I always use this when baking or making smoothies.

- Canned wild tuna in water or canned wild Pacific salmon - great fast protein to add to a salad

- Tins of sardines and kippers (our kids eat these for after school snack, on top of any lunch salad, or post workout meal)

- Organic, sulfite free sundried tomatoes

- Jars of organic crushed tomatoes (no sugar—just tomatoes)

- Tea - Green, peppermint or ginger if you like. It's great for digestion and relaxation.

- Organic Que Pasa tortilla chips

- Organic popcorn – air popped

- Brown rice crackers

- Organic dark chocolate chips. Keep them in the freezer for baking or snacking! Makes a great snack with some raw almonds if you're craving chocolate! (Make sure you limit this to no more than a handful of chocolate and almonds at a time.) Organic dark chocolate can be very good for you so watch which chocolate you eat (milk chocolate and white chocolate do not provide the benefits of real chocolate.)

- Raw cacao beans and powder. Great for protein shakes and adding to stuff for an antioxidant boost!

- Nutracleanse: an organic combination of flax seed, psyllium husk, dandelion root powder, burdock root powder, and fenugreek seed powder. We make a quick almond milk porridge with this.

## FOR YOUR FRIDGE

- Lemons. For cooking with, but also you should drink lemon water every morning to help create a "basic" versus acidic balance in your blood.
- Eggs. We eat at least once a week. Make sure they are local, pastured organic eggs.
- Coconut aminos (natural soy free version of soya sauce)
- Unsweetened almond milk (Costco has the best price or make it yourself and save $$)
- Chia and hemp seeds (awesome protein and great fiber)
- Grass Fed butter and Ghee (NO margarine ... EVER ... it's horrible.)
- Fresh vegetables – LOTS and LOTS and LOTS. Your choice, but try to have all colors every day. Examples - spinach/broccoli/red pepper/tomatoes/carrots. We literally just buy what's on sale every time we go because we like them all, but we just choose our favorites and try to eat whatever is in season! Squash, asparagus, zucchini, and yams - it's endless
- Onion and garlic. Needed for flavoring in pretty much everything
- Avocados – one of the best fats you can eat. We always have 2 or 3 on hand because you often have to wait for them to ripen. Great on salads or for making guacamole.

- Fruit!! Lots!! Treat yourself to stuff you love. Eat it mostly in the mornings; especially fruits like apples/pears/berries/cherries/apricots/bananas ... just buy what's in season!

- Any fresh herbs. We usually only buy one at a time because they spoil fast. For example, we love basil so we always buy it and chop it up on everything, especially salad dressings. It is also very easy to grow herbs in your windowsill and it will save you some money.

- Salmon - wild Pacific, or halibut (buy at your local Fishmonger -best prices and freshest fish)

- Grass fed organic beef, bison, turkey, chicken - no injected antibiotics or hormones whatsoever!

- Natural Factors Acidophilus Capsules

- Honegar- bottle of raw apple cider vinegar and raw honey – best in salad dressings, or add to sparkling water for a natural healthy 'pop'.

## DO NOT BUY!

- Anything that says "white enriched flour" or "hydrogenated" in the ingredients

- Bottled salad dressings. Most of them are full of creams, bad oils, and sugars (there are a few good ones out there, but you can simply make your own faster and better!)

- Margarine – it's horrible for you – just try to read the ingredients.

- Hot dogs and Kraft dinner

- Pop - not ever. Especially diet pop as it contains

aspartame which is a neurological toxin known to contribute to causing cancer, diabetes, Alzheimer's disease and obesity

- Juice-- check out the sugar content-you will be surprised that many have the same content as Coca-Cola

- Anything with MSG, high fructose corn syrup, aspartame, nitrates, or artificial colorings or flavorings. These are completely off limits!

- Basically anything processed or packaged. It's not worth it and it's not the way God made it!

That is our "general" grocery list. So, of course you don't have to buy all of this at once. Start by adding into your cupboards some of the good stuff – or go "full out" and get rid of all the dysfunctional stuff and start fresh![63]

## MEAL PLANNING

The key to successfully making *any* diet change is to have a comprehensive list of food you can eat…that you actually want to eat. Focus on what you can have, and not what you can't have.

In our home, I spend 30 minutes on Sunday nights planning our meals for the week. We have special traditions in our family and every Friday night, we have "Pizza Movie Night". My husband makes a homemade spelt or almond flour pizza crust, homemade sauce, and adds a variety of toppings. Once it is ready, our family enjoys a hot pizza watching a family movie. We have been doing this for 8 years and counting. Another tradition we implement, is that every Sunday night is our 'games night' where we have a meal and then after clean up, we all sit down as a family and play a board game.

We also have 'theme' days, to help keep things flowing

throughout the week. For example, every Thursday night is typically 'Asian" inspired cuisine. Wednesdays is "Fish", Tuesdays is Italian, and Sundays are either Mexican, or barbecue (if it is summertime). From there, I can create a nice variety of foods based around the theme.

You can download your FREE copy of a meal plan at drjodycox.com.


## THE NEXT STEP

If you are still feeling overwhelmed at making some new changes, then start with making green Smoothies. They are very nutritious and easy to digest and will immediately start getting some good nutrients into your body. Don't go crazy too much fruit as it can be taxing on your body. A good balanced smoothie consists of 60% organic greens, 30% good quality fat (like coconut oil, or half an avocado), 10% ripe fruit and nuts. They are awesome for your entire family--and affordable too! Buy ripe fruit on sale and then freeze it. Kale, spinach, parsley are so easy to grow in your backyard making it easy on your budget. They are loaded with healthy minerals (e.g. calcium and iron) and vitamins. And most importantly, they are alkalizing which helps with weight loss, prevents osteoporosis and increases energy! Leafy greens also contain chlorophyll, which resembles human blood-like a healthy blood transfusion. Mix it up by adding a handful of frozen cranberries or blueberries. Cinnamon is a nice sweet addition (just 1/2 teaspoon of cinnamon per day can lower LDL cholesterol, boosts cognitive function and memory, helps relieve arthritis pain, and has a regulatory effect on blood sugar).

Smoothies in our family are enjoyed mainly as an afterschool snack or a lunch. I also recommend them as a 'reboot' for people who are doing a health cleanse or healing from an illness. They are also handy for those times when you are running behind schedule in the morning and need something nutritious to get into everyone. Plus, it is a great way to get those nutritious raw greens into our kids when they might not necessarily be excited to eat some kale just yet.

One last word about smoothies—they are meant to replace a meal, not complement it. If you took everything you put in a smoothie and put it on a plate in front of you and ate it, you would be full, right? So that is your meal. They are just another way to enjoy a bunch of really healthy food and make it highly nutritious and easily digestible. Please note that I don't suggest that smoothies become your everyday meal. There are plenty of other amazing nutrient dense foods to enjoy, like good quality meats and other vegetables and this should be your regular dietary routine. However, smoothies are a healthy good start to introduce some quality easily digestible high fiber foods into your body as you begin to make changes. In the last part of this book, you will find delicious smoothie recipes.

## TIPS FOR ENJOYING SMOOTHIES

We are always asked about what type of smoothie to make, what type of blender to use, and where to get the produce to make it affordable. Keeping in mind that our findings are based on years from our personal experience and backed up with research from multiple resources, here is what we have found.

When you are just getting started on trying on smoothies, the Magic Bullet is an affordable option (approximately $30) and does a great job. We used this for two years and found it to be amazing, but as the kids grew older, we needed something more powerful and bigger for the family. Plus by that time, we had committed to making smoothies on a regular basis, so it made sense to go to the next level.

Best all-around blender: Blendtec. I swear, this will change your life! It is super powerful and will blend, chop, or whip anything into a juice or smoothie, or make wholesome sugar free nut milks and butters! It has a low oxidization rate which simply means that less oxidization, less free radical exposure, more purity in your produce, and better for your blood cells. It also fits on your countertop. That was a big determiner for me as opposed to the Vita-mix. These are pricey, so if you are just getting started with smoothies, I suggest buy a Magic Bullet, then once you determine that you are going to be making smoothies more often, invest in a Blendtec. (Side note: I have heard that these are now sold in Costco) www.blendtec.com

Smoothies can be enjoyed and stored in large Mason jars. You can also purchase cool white plastic lids (BHA free) that fit onto any mason jar, and avoid the tinkering of the metal ring and lids. I have cut my finger too many times on the metal lids.

The key to enjoy smoothies are straws. If you have kids or fussy people, you can serve a smoothie with a straw. It is easy to consume, and you don't have to fuss with all that 'smoothie' stuff getting on your lips and giving you an unwanted moustache. The best straws are stainless steel straws which are easy to clean. They are cost effective, and you will never feel guilty about throwing out copious amounts of straws ever again.

## WHAT TYPE OF ALMOND MILK TO BUY AND WHERE TO GET IT

Homemade almond milk is super easy, has no preservatives or sugars, and is much kinder on the grocery budget. Here's how:

## HOMEMADE ALMOND MILK

Simply soak 1 cup of almonds with a pinch of salt overnight, then rinse in the morning.

Add 4 cups of cold water.

Throw into a high speed blender for 30 seconds.

Strain through a Nut Milk bag into a large bowl.

Transfer to a large Mason jar and store in fridge.

A Nut Milk bag is a micro-mesh straining bag, found at grocery stores and can be used repeatedly. Simple!

If we have to buy almond milk, we buy unsweetened almond milk. You can use nut milk in place of regular milk – in cooking, baking, smoothies, coffee & tea, and of course on your breakfast cereal.

# YOUR **EAT TO THRIVE** CHECKLIST

- **Eat whole foods first.** If it comes in a package, it probably isn't a whole food. You will save yourself a lot of time and money by shopping the perimeter of the grocery store—buying fresh quality produce.

- **Cut out excessive sugar.** In fact, just do a major overhaul in your cupboards and pantry and throw out anything that is refined sugar (white, brown, high fructose corn syrup), looks like sugar, or has labels on it that you can't even read.

- **Get Fat!** Don't worry, you won't actually get fat from eating quality fats. In fact, you will burn body fat by eating and cooking with quality fats. Best fats are avocados, coconut oil, ghee (or clarified butter) and macadamia nuts.

- **Cut out** processed flours and if you can, **reduce** your grains.

- **Source out** local fresh eggs, a local fishmonger, and a local butcher for organic grass fed meats

- Spend 10 minutes at the end of the week **meal planning** for 7 days.

- Most importantly---above all—**SHUT DOWN and SIT UP** when you are having a meal, so that you can be present and intentional with your food—it is for your enjoyment and nourishment.

# Chapter 8: Sleep to Rejuvenate

Did you know your body heals while you are sleeping? Sleep is more important than most people realize. During sleep, the brain does some 'house cleaning' and memory is increased. Research shows that lack of proper sleep leads to all sorts of dis-eases, from difficulty concentrating, weight gain, and depression.[64] Lack of proper sleep can even lead to brain shrinkage and Alzheimer's disease.

## WHAT IS THE BEST TIME FOR SLEEP?

"Early to bed, early to rise, makes you strong, healthy and wise", is absolutely true. Getting to bed before 11 p.m. is a best practice followed by the healthiest, most energized people in the world. [65] [66] However, this can vary due to your age and occupation. Clearly, babies need more sleep than adults, and some adults are in careers that involve night shifts and simply cannot physically get to bed early.

It really comes down to complete sleep cycles. During the night, your sleep follows a predictable pattern, moving back and forth between deep restorative sleep (non-REM) and dreaming (REM sleep). During the deep restorative stages of sleep, the body repairs and regrows tissues, builds bone and muscle, and strengthens the immune system. During the dreaming stage, your brain is more active, and your heart rate and breathing quickens. [67] Together, these stages combined form a complete sleep cycle. Each cycle typically lasts about 90 minutes and repeats four to six times over the course of a night. The way it works is the earlier you go to bed, the more restorative sleep stages you get. The later you go to bed, the less restorative sleep which means you find yourself waking up feeling like you 'didn't have a good sleep'.[68]

Even if you've enjoyed a full night's sleep, getting out of bed can be difficult if your alarm goes off when you're in the middle of deep sleep. If you want to make mornings less painful, or if you know you only have a limited time for sleep, then try setting a wake-up time that's a multiple of 90 minutes which is the length of the average sleep cycle. For example, if you go to bed at 10 p.m., set your alarm for 5:30 (a total of 7 ½ hours of sleep) instead of 6:00 or 6:30. You may feel more refreshed at 5:30 than with another 30 to 60 minutes of sleep because you're getting up at the end of a sleep cycle when your body and brain are already close to wakefulness.

Lastly, there are several great apps you can download to help you fall asleep quicker and deeper. My personal favourite is Pzizz. It's free and it works. I use it when I travel or have jet lag.

## GREAT POSTURE POSITIONS FOR A DEEP SLEEP

Misaligned vertebrae and tight muscles can lead to an uncomfortable and shallow sleep which will leave you feeling groggy in the morning. Not only that, but your sleeping style at night can lead to health problems in the morning. Here are the optimal positions for a healthy sleep and the ones to avoid:

BEST: On your back

Sleeping on your back ensures proper circulation to the brain, maintains your back and neck in a neutral position, and also helps to reduces acid reflux.

GOOD: On your side

Side sleepers, you're doing it right and left side is best. In addition to side sleeping which helps to reduce snoring, sleeping on one's left side also eases heartburn and acid reflux, making it easier to fall and stay asleep. It's a great option during pregnancy too, when back sleeping puts too much pressure on the spine. Make sure you pull your head and pillow back so that your neck is not curled in. This allows to a neutral spinal position which helps to take tension off your spine and spinal cord.

BAD: In the fetal position

It may feel comfy, but sleeping with your body curved in the fetal position restricts breathing and compresses vital organs. In addition, it places a tensile stress on the length of your spinal cord.

WORST: On your stomach

Spending seven to nine hours a night sleeping stomach-down with your head and neck turned to one side or the other is asking for trouble. Try walking all day with your head turned to one side only. I bet by the end of the day, you will have a sore neck! Same case when you are sleeping on your tummy. You might be feeling it in the morning with a stiff neck or headache but it also puts stress on joints and muscles, leading to nerve irritation, pain, tingling and numbness. This position flattens the natural neck curve and will lead to degeneration and arthritis over time.

FINAL TIP: Pillow-supplemented sleep

Regardless of which sleeping position you prefer, it's highly likely that you can get better night's rest with less pain in the morning by supporting your body with a pillow. Side sleepers can place a pillow between their knees, which prevent twisting on the low back and hips, and allows for a neutral spine. For your head and neck, we recommend Align-Right Pillows as they not only provide for an amazing sleep, but also facilitate a healthy curve in your neck!

## ROUTINE FOR SLEEP

**Prepare ahead**

By preparing ahead, packing your lunch, setting out your clothes or creating a to-do list, you'll set yourself up for success and not have to rush in the morning, leaving time for other things.

**Set the scene**

Turn off the screens an hour or two before bed. Smartphones, laptops, computers, TVs and tablets all emit melatonin-disrupting blue light directly into our staring, transfixed eyeballs.

Eliminate, remove, or cover up any sources of light in your bedroom, even the tiny blinking ones. Blackout blinds over your windows, duct tape over your blinking lights, and towels under doors may be warranted to achieve true darkness.

Make sure your room is cool and open a window. Studies show that the optimal room temperature for sleep is quite cool, between 60 to 68 degrees F (15.5 to 20 C). Keeping your room too hot can lead to restless sleep.[69]

Music is also great to cue your body for a routine sleep. One of the best songs to begin this process is called "Weightless" by Marconi Union. It is calibrated at a frequency that slows down your heartbeat and prepares your body for rest. You can pick it up on iTunes for a mere $1.29.

**Nurture your body for nighttime.**

Magnesium just before bed, can help you get to sleep faster and deeper. Magnesium is a naturally occurring mineral in your body that circulates predominately in your bones, but also in your organs and muscle tissue. Many studies point out that environmental stress, emotional stress, and physical stress will contribute to a decrease in the body's natural magnesium content. We take a citrate form of magnesium drink and enjoy this nightcap about 30 minutes before bed after an active or stressful day. We enjoy Natural Calm Magnesium powder.

**Make a nourishing nightcap.**

You can end the evening with a bedtime tonic sans alcohol and caffeine, perhaps right in your bed. Enjoy some warm water with lemon, ginger (helps with digestion), chamomile tea, warm almond milk with vanilla powder and cinnamon, or a turmeric ginger tea which is very comforting and healing.

# WRITE A TO-FEEL LIST RATHER THAN A TO- DO LIST

To-do lists are overwhelming, and in my opinion are best done at the beginning of the week or at least in the morning, when you are feeling mentally refreshed and on purpose. If you want to feel overwhelmed with intention, excitement, and childlike joy, try ending the evening by writing down how you want to feel the following day. Just write down the first word that comes to mind: loved, supported, happy, joyful, productive, spirited, intuitive, and forgiven. It will give you a sense of anticipation and can create a purposeful next day.

## TEACHING YOUR KIDS TO SLEEP

Kids' brains and bodies are constantly working; growing bones, developing muscles (with all that play), and making new nervous system connections in their growing brains. When you really stop to think just how dependent newborns are and then add in all the growth and development that go through into their first year of life, it's very hard work! And all this extra work means that children need a lot more sleep than adults.

If your child does not sleep well, or still appears tired after a reasonable amount of sleep, then there may be underlying issues. High levels of spinal cord tension and the presence of misalignments in the spine can restrict movement, stress the nervous system and even cause pain. Chiropractic adjustments can help your child to relax, fall asleep more easily and sleep longer. [70] Remember good sleep helps to develop memory and alertness and also strengthens the immune system.

# Chapter 9: Take Care of Your Soul

*"I pray that you prosper in ALL things and be in Health just as your soul prospers"*
*- 3 John 1:2*

*"We are a soul with a body,*
*not a body with a soul"*
*-C.S. Lewis*

## QUIT STRIVING!

"If I do this .....then I will...."

You may say to yourself, "If I just eat only organic food, vegan and gluten free, then I will never die from a heart attack." That is just purely false. Because even though, yes-good eating habits will certainly help prevent heart disease and many other ailments, ultimately, it leads to a dangerous and dogmatic belief that you are in total control. Things happen to even the healthiest people on the planet. It necessitates the reminder that you are not in total control. I believe God is. He created you, knows everything about you, and even knows when you will die. It can be a humbling reality, but being humble about your destiny allows you the grace to quit trying to be perfect, and truly enjoy the miracles and moments in life.

That being said, I believe you are alive for a reason, and given a body and a purpose here on earth for God's glory. What you do with your life and body is how you honor God with the gifts He gave you. That might mean that you need to get in shape, or eat better, or have a better financial budget, so that you can be more effective in your life.

## MORNING TIME

*"Be still, and know that I am God"*
*- Psalm 46:10*

Morning time is the best time to get prepared, physically, mentally and spiritually for the day ahead. It sets the pace for your day ahead. Most often this vital time of peace is neglected. Typically people awaken, jump out of bed, scramble to get their breakfast and get going with their day. They then feel overwhelmed, scattered, or disconnected with the day itself. By getting up 1 -2 hours earlier while the rest of the world is sleeping, you will find it like a multivitamin for your soul. Find a place of inspiration in your home, grab a cup of tea and get comfy. You can reflect on your past blessings, or take time to pray, dream, or visualize your day. It can be anything as long as it doesn't involve any Internet, or media that would distract you from being present in this special time. For me, this is the time where I become 'still' and get connected with God in a personal way and then take that feeling to into the presence of my day ahead.

I have trained myself to get up 1-2 hours before the routine of preparing breakfast, showering and getting on with the day. I'll admit, it has taken some time and much discipline to get up so early, but when I do, that preparation in my heart transcends throughout the rest of my day, and it can do the same for you too.

Some people say that they are just 'not a morning person' but just haven't given it a try — or they've gotten up an hour or two earlier all at once, and hated being so tired. This is why it is so important to make the changes gradually — it's not that you're not a morning person, it's just that you tried to change too quickly and are suffering. There are two other major lifestyle factors that could be preventing you from getting up early. You may be eating sugary or high carbohydrate foods late at night and not allowing proper digestion and digestive rest to take place. Or you are just going to bed way too late. You need to be in bed with the lights out by 10:30pm folks! By just changing your late night eating habits and going to bed early, you will naturally begin to wake up earlier feeling much more well rested! Just try it.

The best method for changing the time you wake up is to do it gradually — 15 minutes earlier for 2-4 days, until you feel used to it, and then repeat until you come to the time you would like to wake up at. If you get up at 8 a.m. normally, don't suddenly change it to 6 a.m. Try 7:45 a.m. first. Here is how:

1. **Get excited.** The night before, think of one thing you'd like to do in the morning that excites you. It could be something you want to write, or a new running route, spending some quiet time with God, or something you'd like to read, or a work project that's got you fired up. In the morning, when you wake up, remember that exciting thing, and that will help motivate you to get up.

2. **Jump out of bed.** Yes, jump out of bed. With enthusiasm and gratitude. Jump up and spread your arms wide as if to say,

"Yes! Thank God, I am alive! Ready to see what exciting things are going happen today." Seriously, it works.

3. **Put your alarm across the room.** If it's right next to you, you'll hit the snooze button. So put it on the other side of the room, so you'll have to get up (or jump up) to turn it off. Then, get into the habit of going straight to the bathroom once you've turned it off. Once you're finished in the bathroom, you're much less likely to go back to bed. At this point, remember your exciting thing. If you didn't jump out of bed, at least stretch your arms wide and greet the day.


## PRAYER & GRATITUDE

*"Do not be anxious about anything, but in every situation, by prayer and petition, with thanksgiving, present your requests to God."*
*Philippians 4:6*

Prayer is powerful, and it connects you with a purpose for all that is going on in your life. Even if you don't know God, you can still spend time contemplating all the things you are thankful for. Ann Voskamp, author of One Thousand Gifts, puts it best when she says, "Joy is a function of gratitude, and gratitude is a function of perspective. You only begin to change your life when you begin to change the way you see." A great place to start is just taking time reflecting on the top 10 things you are grateful for right now. In fact, studies show that people who feel grateful, on average, have lower stress levels, lower blood pressure, more satisfying relationships, higher grades, smoke less, get in fewer arguments, feel a stronger sense of communication and are more likely to donate money or volunteer their time.[71]

## JOURNALING

> *"The pen is mightier than the sword."*
> *~Edward Bulwer-Lytton*

Every year, I finish a journal and begin a new one. My journal is another 'legacy gift' to my family when I am no longer here on earth. I keep my dreams in it, write down events that have had an impact on my life, gratitude moments, reflections, and sometimes I will tape a cherished letter or card in it. Furthermore, research shows that journaling your life's experiences is one of the most effective strategies to cope with stress.[72]

Find a journal that lays flat on a table. Get a nice pen and keep your journal handy at all times. By actively writing you will experience more clarity of thought and revelation. When you reflect upon your past journal entries, you may see answered prayers, or a whole new appreciation for the things you had gone through in the past. You might even find something you wrote two years ago that now serves a greater meaning in your current situation.

## MUSIC

> *"The atmosphere of expectation is the*
> *breeding ground for miracles."*
> *— Israel Houghton*

Music is a major influence in our life. My husband plays guitar, harmonica, banjo and recently, enjoyed learning the ukulele. Our kids both take piano lessons, and we constantly love making music and dancing to it. In the morning time, I will set the stage with waking up the children to light inspirational tunes. Listening to or performing music helps to stimulate the auditory cortex of the right brain and leads to increased creativity.

You can try playing light forgiving songs as we wind down the day. Hawaii ocean waves are amazing to help unwind. Music also helps to create an atmosphere for healing.

> *"Music opens doors and music stimulates the brain…. It's a wonderful applicable skill that only makes you a more capable human"*
> *- Chris Hadfield, Canadian Astronaut*

## FORGIVE

There is a great quote saying that 'the root of all sin is in lack of forgiveness.' Forgiveness can be a touchy topic for so many people, including me. It often requires the act of grace. Grace is unmerited favor, or forgiving someone that doesn't deserve to be forgiven. If you have identified unresolved forgiveness, and need help to take those steps—there are many ways of forgiving the offender. It can be a letter, email or in person. If you feel you need more help on it, then certainly seek counsel. Every time I have forgiven someone for something, I instantly experience freedom. Most people will admit that pride stops them from forgiving someone. When I first heard that, it stopped me in my tracks because I realized I had more of a 'pride' issue than a 'forgiveness' issue. All I can say is if you are reading this, and are starting to feel skittish, then maybe that is a direction that you need to explore during your healing process.

From a physical perspective, here are some amazing health benefits that forgiveness can lead to:

- Healthier relationships
- Greater spiritual and psychological well-being
- Less anxiety, stress and hostility
- Lower blood pressure
- Fewer symptoms of depression
- Lower risk of alcohol and substance abuse

As you let go of grudges, you'll no longer define your life by how you've been hurt. You don't have to forget it, but you can forgive. In the process, you might even find compassion and understanding.


## BE BRAVE

*"It's my belief that true fearlessness comes from living loved..."*
*- Sarah Bessey*


I often hear people say how they wish or would like to own a flower shop, or run a half marathon, or become a teacher or .....(fill in the blank), but .... All too often that statement lingers out in space and then dies down, again. We become comfortable cowards and settle for our cozy mediocrity. This happens to me too. However, I have learned that fear does not come from God. For the most part fear is something that is made up, created in our minds to self-sabotage us from truly reaching our potential.

The only way to conquer fear is to step through it. Easier said than done, right? I'm not talking about just launching into something just on a whim or a response from social pressure. I'm talking about discerning the difference between the anxiety that comes from doing the wrong thing, and the good butterflies that come when you are braving the new right thing.

It's all about the next step—even if it is just a baby step. Every time you take that uneasy, uncomfortable step, you will find that----hey, you are actually, 'OK'. We call it "Stepping into the Gap" meaning the uncomfortable zone of where transformation begins. One of my mentors and coaches, Dr. Marie Geschwandtner, of Warrior Coaching explains, "the Gap is where life happens."

I love what author and blogger, Sarah Bessey goes on to address her perspective of bravery in saying:

"It's about daring to be honest with our own self, of laying down our excuses or justifications or disguises, of asking ourselves what we really want, of forgiveness, of honesty, of choosing the hard daily work of restoration, of staying resolutely alive when everyone else is just numbing themselves against life."

The way I am able to take the next step into my fears is by looking back at my life and reflecting on all those situations of uncertain times and seeing how I did get through it. I can look back to see that God has 'had my back' all this time and will certainly never fail me. When I chose to take the 'road less traveled', I always experienced transformation and exhilaration, and you will too!

So take a moment to think about what is holding you back:

*What is it that you need to speak into, or take an action step into?*

And then look back at your life and think about those courageous moments where you actually did something you didn't think you could do. How did you feel? I am assuming you survived, and quite possibly, it made a difference in your life. It is time to jump in again!

## BE GENEROUS

*"We make a living by what we get, but we make a Life by what we give"*
*-Winston Churchill*

True generosity is described as going over the top while having no guarantee of a reward. Generosity is not about what you can gain if you give; it is all about just simply giving. No matter what little resources, not just our money but also many other things such as our time, we all have the ability to be generous.

We shouldn't be generous because we feel obliged. If we are feeling pressured to do something but don't have the time, it's ok to say no. But that 'no' or 'yes' shouldn't be filled with contempt or guilt.

We shouldn't be generous just to receive recognition. We should do it out of the goodness of our heart and because we genuinely want to, without any ulterior motives.

There is a reason why discontented people have a hard time giving. Can you find the word "miser' in the word miserable? On the other hand, spontaneous acts of generosity can be a quick way to snap you out of your funk and put you back on track. Generosity goes hand in hand with contentment, in that the more content you are, the easier it is to give, and in return, the more content you become. In other words, the more we give away, the more 'richer' we become.

# Chapter 10: Belong to a Life Group

## FIND YOUR PEOPLE

Let's face it, loneliness sucks. I heard this great comment about health and community and it goes like this:

*The "I" in illness is isolation*
*The "W" in wellness is we*

Vancouver is the second biggest city in Canada and rated as one of the most beautiful cities in the world. Recently, it was reported that it has the highest rate of social media usage in North America. Yet, it is also reported that it has the highest rate of loneliness. [73] Social technology is perceived to make us feel more connected when in reality we are experiencing more disconnect within our community.

For this reason alone, it is so important to connect with each other by being physically present. Make an effort to connect in churches, schools, work, exercise classes, art courses, sports groups, gardening socials, and volunteering. Quit hiding behind your computer or iPhone and look up. There are fabulous people waiting to meet you.

# YOUR CIRCLE OF INFLUENCE

*"Show me your friends, and I will show you your future"*

Our circle of influence guides our decisions we make. Relationship is the currency of all reality. Take time to evaluate your family's philosophy on health, core values and vision. If you are a parent, just ask yourself: whom do you want to mentor your kids? Then take a look at whom you let into your inner circle of influence. Hang out with people that have a similar vision to you and are moving in the same direction.

Who is your Support in Crisis?

I learned a vital lesson this week from a crisis that happened to me a few days ago. Our family cat, Noel was on our doorstep from his morning jaunt and I saw that his right eye was sealed shut with fluid running from it. Being new with cats, I was shocked and not quite sure what to do. I held him and looked into his eye--I couldn't see blood or a scratch. He was meowing and you could tell he was uncomfortable. About 20 minutes later, it was getting worse and his eye has completely swollen up to the point that all I can see is a pink membrane covering his entire eye!! What do I do? Is this cat going blind? At first I panicked not knowing whether I should rush the cat to the vet. Who should I call? So out of intuition, I bundled him up and brought him to the one place where I knew I would get the calm support that I instantly needed--my clinic. After being comforted by my team, who knew my core values; I was clear to regain the truth that I have always known.... that just like us, our cat was going to heal on his own.

So I did the one thing I knew that would help him instantly-

-adjusted his spine to tone his nervous system.

I adjusted his atlas (the first cervical vertebra where a massive amount of nerves sit controlling major functions such as the eyes, ears, nose and throat).

Within 10 minutes, his eye started to resolve almost completely back to normal! No joke.

This lesson made me think how easy it is to fall into a panic when you are in a crisis--with your kids, your friends, or even yourself. The outcome will be determined by your core belief AND who you have in your support group. Those people who truly know you and will be there to calm you down, affirm you, speak the truth to you, and re-align you with your core values once again.

## SPEAKING LIFE

*"The tongue has the power of life and death.."*
*-Proverbs 18:21*

Speaking Life is about verbalizing powerful and affirming words into the heart. These words can be so transformational that when you speak life, you cast away fears and anxieties and restore internal confidence.

When my Dad was awaiting his quadruple bypass surgery, the days I spent pre and post operation were a great learning experience for me. The care that my Dad received at the Kelowna General Hospital was exceptional in every way. I felt like all the nurses had all gone to cheerleading school before they actually became nurses. The cardiac team was so encouraging and joyful and I believe that was a huge part of my Dad's speedy recovery. It taught me a great lesson on speaking life into people despite the circumstances. It was not a denial of the reality, but speaking positive affirmations into sorrowful situations can restore hope and perseverance. It truly changed the atmosphere in the entire room. What would it be like if we all had to go to a cheerleading school as a requirement to work and serve, or be a parent?

In our children's rooms we have these giant size prints hanging above their beds that we custom created with In-Nate Prints. They are the life giving words that we want to speak over our kids so that every night they are strengthened and affirmed of who we believe they are. You can create a poster or a picture for your child or loved one to remind them of who they truly are created to be. This is a powerful tool that you can use to cue yourself to speak into their lives.

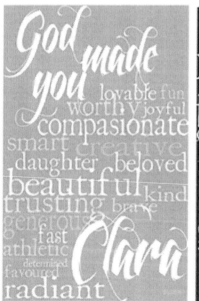 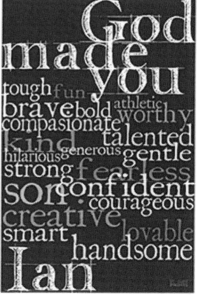

# Chapter 11: Dream Big

*"No matter where you are at, you have a greater potential than you think you have."*
-Dr. Jody Cox

## WHAT IS YOUR GIFT?

*"Each of us should use whatever gifts he has received to serve others, faithfully administrating God's grace in various forms."*
*-1 Peter 4: 10-11*

There is a uniqueness in each of us—life is a gift that you have been given. Whether you have the gift to be a speaker, a musician, or a hairdresser, use your talent to make this world a better place.

The way to identify your gift is to actually examine what your major weakness is. This is quite the opposite of what you might expect to hear. Take a moment to ponder what is your breaking point--the thing that brings you to your knees or stops you in your tracks. The thing that you don't like to admit or shudder to think about. Typically, once you figure out what that is, you can look at the exact opposite of that belief and you will find your strength or gift. For example, my weakness is that sometimes, I can feel unvalued and stupid. That feeling comes from my past of not feeling valued as a child. I would often struggle and default to self-sabotage when opportunities arose for taking on roles of leadership. However, once I finally identified my wound, I was able to see the actual gift inside me, because the opposite of invaluable is--priceless. And I know that that is actually my true calling—that I am an immensely valuable person and my gift is the ability to bring new hope. And when I do step into my calling, my gift--then lives change for the better.

So take some time to meditate on where your weaknesses are. It is not that hard. Just begin by reflecting this past week on what things you said or didn't say that you regretted. Or ask yourself what did you hold back from doing? And then ask yourself why you held back, or why you said what you said. What were you afraid of? Or fill in the blank: "The reason I did what I did is because I felt (unworthy/ stupid/ unattractive/_".
The more specific and the deeper you go, the more clear your answer will be. You might feel pretty vulnerable doing this process, but stick with it until you have clarity.

Then, once you find your weakness, look to the opposite strength— and there, you will find your gift, your true identity. Write it down in your journal. Now. You should experience that 'warm fuzzy feeling' or good butterflies when you look at what you have written down. That is who you are! And once you find your calling, you are ready for the next step— time to dream!

# BEGIN BY DREAMING

*"For I know the plans I have for you,"*
*declares the LORD, "plans to prosper you*
*and not to harm you, plans to give you hope*
*and a future."*
*-Jeremiah 29:11*

If you are feeling washed up, it is likely that you took a dream and placed it aside to do something else. Maybe your something 'else' was a job that paid the bills instead of pursuing the passion that you have inside you. Whatever it is, if you've placed that dream aside I can guarantee it's affecting you, your health and everyone around you MORE than you realize. The solution? Allow yourself the pleasure of dreaming again. You were born to dream.

If you need some inspiration, then get outside with nature. Look around at all of the Earth's beautiful surrounding. Listen to some inspirational music, or watch an inspiring documentary, or flip through a travel magazine. This can be tough for many people who have become skeptical or feel jaded from past experiences and now have a hard time dreaming again.

**Time to Dream On!**

Here are some questions to get you started on discovering your unique purpose. Take a few minutes to write out your answers.

What would you like to be?

What would you like to do?

What would you like to have?

If things worked out exactly the way you want, what would be different?

You may not have revelation right now, but you are starting to exercise the process of discovering the depths of whom you are, especially if you understand your gift.

*"When there is no vision, the people perish"*
*- Proverbs 29:18*

## WRITE IT OUT

Begin with the end in mind. Write a letter to yourself ten years from now, and lay it out large - all of your biggest dreams and goals. If you don't have a family and you want children, write that letter to your unborn child 10 years from now. The more specific the details, the better.

**Here is my story**

Ten years ago at a seminar in Ottawa, it was minus 30 degrees Celsius and we had to go for a run outside. It was so cold that everyone came back with frozen eyelashes! The focus of that seminar was writing down your dreams and specifically writing a letter to yourself 10 years from now. Many things that I wrote in that letter have actually come true. Here we were in Ottawa, minus 30, and I was writing a letter to my son and daughter who had not been born yet. I wrote that we were living by the ocean, owning our own dream practice, serving a large volume of people, with enough revenue that we could live in a nice home and give to our church, and to the needy within our community and around the world. And now, probably 80% of it has come true. And in fact now 85% by writing this book! This might take a bit of time, but it is well worth it.

# BREAK IT DOWN

Once you have written your future story, review it and identify your dreams within the story. Then categorize these dreams into the following:

- Spiritual
- Family
- Career
- Physical
- Recreational

Once you have written down your dreams in the 5 different categories, the next step is to assign a timeline to each dream. Decide if the dream is:

1. Immediate (can this happen within a month?)
2. This Year (is this something that can happen within this year?)
3. Future Plans (your vision over the next 10 years)

Notice that some of your dreams are really quickly attainable, while others may take a longer time until they are realized. Either way, now you have a fresh overview or 'compass' of your new life. Are you excited yet??!

# VISUALIZATION

*"It's not what you are looking at that matters,
it is what you see"*
*- Henry David Thoreau*

*"For as he thinks in his heart, so is he"*
*-Proverbs 23:7*

For a long time, scientists believed that the brain was static after childhood. It was also believed that genetics was destiny. While most of our DNA (genetic makeup) stays the same during our lives, research now shows that the level of gene expression can be completely altered by experience, perceptions and lifestyle choices. This is called epigenetics. It simply means that your perceptions can control your biology, and thus affect your health.

*Neuroplasticity* is the word for the actual chemical changes that occur within the brain and its cells. What we think, what we learn, what we focus on, and what we do will actually change brain structures for the future, and affect the state of our bodies. There was an interesting study done with two groups where one group did physical exercise over a period of 5 days and the other group visualized doing that exact same exercise over the same period. At the end of the study, the group that did their physical activity improved their muscle strength by 30 percent. The group that just visualized them doing the physical activity increased their muscle strength by 22 percent! [74]

Visualization can be particularly useful when overcoming stressful and anxious situations. For example, you might have a meeting scheduled in the afternoon that you are really nervous about. Taking time to visualize yourself in that meeting and how you want to respond to various scenarios can leave you feeling much more at ease.

In terms of achieving your short and long term goals, once you have your dreams outlined, the next step is to spend time visualizing them coming true. You can do this during your morning time, or schedule a time once a week where you focus on visualizing your dreams coming true.

*"What we think and what we focus on can actually change our brain."*
*-Dr. Caroline Leaf, Neuroscientist*

# Chapter 12: Take Action

*"Success is really tomorrow's result
from today's effort."*

The key to making lasting improvements is setting a goal and sticking with it. This is where the magic happens. Without a goal, there's nothing to work toward. Without a commitment to your goal, you'll never achieve it. But when you combine a clear vision with a strong commitment, there is no obstacle you can't overcome.

Goal Setting can sound overwhelming at first, but once you break it down into chunks of long and short terms goals, it can be really simple. At the same time, you need to cultivate an appreciation for delayed Gratification. Not all goals are achieved in 1 week as some of us would like. That is why is nice to have short-term goals in addition to long-term goals. The next step is to take your Dream Categories (long and short term), and begin to outline a step-by-step process.

## TAKE YOUR DREAMS AND TURN THEM INTO ACTION STEPS

*"Action trumps knowledge. Discipline trumps
talent. Implementation trumps intention."*

Ask yourself this:

If you knew that every action step you take impacts your life and the life of others; what would you do differently?

If this change were easy, would you want to make it?

What makes it hard?

Sometimes, we get overwhelmed at projects and then just simply put them off. But by taking the very next step, it makes it easier to do. Everyone has their own type of yearly planner, calendar, iCal, or day timer. The next step is to take your Dream Categories (long and short term), and begin to outline a step by step process until you have completed that goal.

For example, let's say you have a short term goal of running your first 10 Km race. Here is what a 10-step outline might look like:

Step 1: Look for a race within the next 3 months.

Step 2: Register for the race.

Step 3: Buy running shoes.

Step 4: Download a 10-week running schedule and print it out. Enter your running plan into your weekly schedule.

Step 5: Begin running plan.

Step 6: Find someone for accountability.

Step 7: Pick up race kit day before race.

Step 8: Have race day gear ready.

Step 9: Have race day nutrition planned and ready.

Step 10: Run the 10K race.

Voila! See how easy that was? You can break it down into manageable and realistic chunks, and then it certainly doesn't seem to hard anymore.

Once you have your steps outlined, put each step into each week of your calendar. That way, each week, you are taking another step in the right direction. Before you know it, you will have accomplished your goal!

## STICK TO THE 'PLAN'

*"You miss 100% of the shots you don't take"*
*-Wayne Gretzky*

How can you get your life in a position to train for your dreams? A lot of times, people will make a resolution like "This year, I am going to take a family trip" or "I'm going to lose 20 pounds" or "I'm going to make more money." Of course this all sounds nice, but the question is, do you have a plan in place for you to make this happen?

The difference between your wishes and actually attaining them is how fully committed you are to the process. Think about it. Are you fully committed towards making a change? Or are you 'half in' and just wishing? Commitment doesn't have to be overwhelming. It just takes an action plan and implementation, step by step, until to reach your goal. If you are feeling stuck, then go back to revisit your dreams. Meditate on your "Big WHY? And then get back on it. If you don't have an actual training schedule in your weekly routine, the chance of any of your resolutions actually coming into fruition are next to nil.

# HOW BIG IS YOUR BUT?

Okay, so this is a question you definitely DON'T want to ask your spouse or friend without further explanation. On paper, however, it is a vital key to revealing what is holding you back. We've all had that moment. A decision or opportunity arises in our life - a new job, a potential relationship, a big move, basically anything that involves some RISK and FAITH. To jump on this opportunity we have to act, and act quickly, or the chance will be lost. So what do you do? Do you follow your heart because you know that it's a good decision yet full of uncertainties. Or do you ponder, think long and hard, and weigh carefully the pros and cons over days, weeks, months, until the opportunity passes? In other words, do you sit on your "but"?

Recently, I had such a decision. I was training over the summer and felt in my heart that I wanted to run a marathon. I had never run so far in my life and don't even consider myself a real runner. I had run half marathons before, but never a full 42km marathon. So my thoughts were - "I can run 21km, BUT could I run 42km?" "I can sign up, BUT what if I can't finish?" or "What if I start the race BUT something goes
wrong and I get injured or worse?" "Other people are real runners, BUT am I? "- on and on it went.

In spite of all of these thoughts and doubts, I knew deep down in my heart that I could do it. I knew it would be grueling, tough, full of pain - and that was okay.

So I took a huge leap of FAITH, signed up and

began to train. I committed to the process. I got off my big "but" and acted!

Guess what? I finished my first marathon. It was indeed grueling, tough, and full of pain - BUT I did it! And I'm so glad I did.

Be aware of what is holding you back from following your heart. Are you full of doubt? Are you not sure if you have what it takes? Is your "But" really holding you back from your true potential? From what I have experienced in my life, and from the transformations I have seen in my patients' lives over the past 17 years, I see that the BEST decisions are made when we follow our heart, not our "but".

- Excerpt from Dr. Ron Pashkewych

Lastly, human tradition focuses on the thing we are trying to accomplish, the habit we are trying to start, or stop. But instead, focus on the process, how far you have already come, and celebrate the journey along the way. Embrace the process with obedience and eventually you will experience the realization of your dreams being fulfilled!

## TOP 3 STRATEGIES FOR SUSTAINABLE CHANGE

1. **Shut down and Sit up**: Shut down all media, phones, buzzes and sounds of phones. Put the newspaper or book away and sit down to IN-JOY your meal. Allow no distraction from you actually connecting your nourishing to your body—so that you can actually enjoy the flavours and *feel* when you are completely satisfied. Try smiling when you are eating. Smiling elevates the nurturing and nourishing aspects of food for your soul.

2.  **Mono-task, not Multi-task:** Chose one thing and do it—and COMPLETE IT! So often we spread our tentacles over everything trying to multi-task. In the quest to accomplish much, we have lost the art of focusing on one thing. We live in a world saturated with multiple messages and images on social media, influences, blogs, tv programs, and even the plethora of self help books. Often well intentioned tasks get sidetracked due to distraction.

    In the end it results in frustration and/or self sabotage. Instead, write down your ONE THING – your one desire—you need to accomplish this week or this year,—thee most important thing—and focus on it. Be intentional with it and do it well.

*"Often he who does too much does too little"*
*– Italian Proverb*

3.  **Own Your Why!** Write down WHY you want to be healthy. I can't say this enough. If you don't have a WHY—all your 'whats' will fall short along the way. Once you have your WHY—write it down and copy it and put it up so you can see it and not get distracted. At the back of this book, is a simple process to help discover your 'Why'. This will be your compass in all your healthy decisions for the year.

*Hope is the ability to hear the music of the future. Faith is the courage to dance to it today!!*

# PART THREE:

## Frequently Asked Questions

## WILL AN ADJUSTMENT HURT?

No, adjustments do not hurt. In fact, it is just the opposite. Many people report that after an adjustment they feel instant relief. Every adjustment is gentle and modified to each patient based on their history and exam findings. Research shows that as a byproduct of an adjustment, endorphins (that "feel good" hormone) are released immediately and that is why so many people say "ahhh" after an adjustment, because it feels so good! What they are experiencing are their nervous system connections being restored.

## WHAT IF I DON'T WANT MY NECK CRACKED? WHAT IS THAT 'POPPING SOUND'?

Don't worry, chiropractors don't want your neck cracked either. Many people think that chiropractors are cracking bones. That is far from the truth. That popping sound is called 'cavitation', and is exactly the same thing that happens when you crack your knuckles. Only that you really aren't cracking anything. It is more of a compression of gases within the joint itself is what you are actually hearing. Now, not every adjustment results in a popping sound and in fact some chiropractic adjusting techniques never cavitate the joint. The goal of an adjustment is to align the spinal joints and take pressure off the nervous system allowing your body to heal better.

Every chiropractor is trained in different techniques to accommodate the patient and deliver the best possible adjustment for that patient based on their history and exam findings. If someone is adverse to hearing that sound, many chiropractors are trained to use a hand held adjusting tool called an Activator or an Integrator instrument to create that same specific and gentle adjustment.

## WHAT DOES IT MEAN TO BE UNDER CHIROPRACTIC CARE?

I heard once you start, you have to keep going. Is that true? No. You don't HAVE to do anything. It is always your choice. We won't make you feel bad if you don't take care of yourself. But think about this analogy: What if all this time you had been brushing your teeth on a daily basis, and one day you just decided to stop brushing your teeth? After all, they look so nice and white, and besides, you don't have any cavities. What do you think would eventually happen? I am suspecting over time and with that kind of poor hygiene, you *would* end up with a cavity, and let's face it - some seriously stinky bad breath!

You brush your teeth on a daily basis because you want to avoid that stinky breath, but more importantly, want to maintain clean healthy teeth. The same applies to wellness chiropractic care. Once we correct your spine to maximum improvement, and then the next goal is to maintain that, so you can function at your best for a lifetime!

As a Chiropractic assistant, I get to witness the many miracles that happen on a daily basis in our clinic. One of our patients, named James, had recently completed his 5 months progress exam. He has been a patient with us over the last six years on and off and would come in for relief care when needed, despite our recommendations to consider corrective chiropractic care, and look to actually improving his current health status.

Five months ago he came back in after we had not seen him in well over a year. By now he was in a lot of pain, depressed and had separated from his wife. We did an exam and took x-rays.

Upon viewing his own x-rays with Dr. Ron, he made a decision that would change his life forever and his journey to corrective chiropractic care began. He works a job with long hours and involves shift work, yet was determined and dedicated to his care.

In fact, he never missed an adjustment. The changes I have seen in him over the past consecutive 5 months have been just amazing. He is glowing, happy and pain free now. We just completed his five month progress exam where another x-ray is taken to see what structural changes have been made in the spine and he had such good progress in that short amount of time.

Besides the incredible results within his physical body, he has got his life back and I am happy to say he has reconciled with his wife! They have just left on a two month trip together where he will continue to do the home spinal correction while away. I look forward to seeing him upon his return and seeing the continued progress in restoring his spine.

- Lauryn, Chiropractic Assistant to New Hope Chiropractic

# HOW OFTEN DO I NEED TO COME SEE YOU?

YOU are the product of accumulation. You didn't get to where you are today from what you did yesterday, or the day the before. You got where you are today from the things you did YEARS ago. It is called a bio- accumulation effect. For instance, if you ate really well for the past 10 years, then your body has definitely been rewarding you. If you decided last week to start eating well after years of neglecting a good healthy diet, then don't get frustrated if you don't feel the results immediately (they will come, but it takes time). If you finally quit smoking, you wouldn't expect your body to just reset itself in a month. Research shows that it takes 20 years until the risk of death from all smoking related causes would be reduced to that of a never-smoker.[75]

Similarly, we would *never ever* make a recommendation for just a couple of adjustments if you have had an accumulation of damage in your spine for years and years.

*"Before I came to New Hope, I was in daily pain that left me tired, irritable, unable to focus and complete daily tasks both at home and at work. I am only 32!*

*Within 6 months of regular chiropractic care at New Hope, I now experience less body pain, better sleep, more energy, more clarity of mind, no headaches, and most of all; I feel happier in general.*

*Thank you Dr. Ron & Dr. Jody"*

*- Tonyia L.*

Based on your exam, posture analysis and x-ray, your Chiropractor will make recommendations for your care.

The goal is to improve the physiology in your spine and nervous system, which thus improves the physiology in your health. So that you can do what you need to do with ease and do what you love to do with effortless energy.

## IF YOUR BODY CAN HEAL ITSELF, THEN WHY WOULD YOU NEED CHIROPRACTIC CARE?

Is this a trick question? Nope. It is true that your body can heal itself. When your spine is in perfect alignment and no stresses are present, then your healing capacity is at its maximum. However, the truth is, life happens, and we all encounter stresses throughout our days which affect our health. These stresses directly affect our spine and nervous system. So even though your body has a tremendous ability to heal, it can't heal optimally if your nervous system is compromised. It would be like straining to see under a dim light. Although you can see, it is not nearly as easy than if the light was fully illuminated. Chiropractic essentially illuminates your light within and helps to counterbalance everyday stresses so your body can work that much better. [76]

Chiropractic is for everybody in the same way that eating good food and exercise is for everybody. It addresses the primary requirement in that for healing to occur—whether you are a newborn or sick and elderly, you have to have optimal nerve and structural function.

## ISN'T CHIROPRACTIC CARE EXPENSIVE?

Absolutely Not! It's all on perspective. First of all, how can you place a value amount on your health? It really comes down to lining up your priorities and values when it comes to deciding how you want to invest your money.

In the long run, taking care of your health now will save you money that you would have to spend later if you were to become unhealthy.

## GETTING WELL AND STAYING WELL IS EXPENSIVE, BUT IT IS CHEAPER THAN BEING SICK

A study tracked the benefit of Wellness Chiropractic care over time (care that follows after your initial correction). They followed 311 chiropractic patients, aged 65 and older, who were under 'maintenance care' for 5 years or longer vs. healthy citizens the same age.

The results showed:

- Chiropractic patients had 50% fewer medical provider visits

- Chiropractic patients had 60.2% fewer hospital admissions

- Chiropractic patients had 59% fewer days hospitalized

- Chiropractic patients had 62% less outpatient surgeries

- Chiropractic patients had 85% less medication costs

In addition, the study found that the chiropractic patients were 60% more likely to be able to keep healthy habit more consistent--that is, when your nerve system is clear of interference; it actually becomes easier for you to maintain healthy habits! [77] [78] [79] [80]

## BEING HEALTHY NOW SAVES YOU MONEY LATER

If you are considering your future financial security, then being healthy pays off. Financial advisor Steve Devlin at

MacDev Financial, shows that healthy people will pay less money on monthly whole life insurance premiums than unhealthy ones. Here are some examples:

---

**40 Year Old Twin Males Need $500,000 of 10 Year Term Life Insurance**

One is a very healthy and fit non-smoker and will only pay $32.40 per month. His twin brother is a smoker and not very healthy. He is overweight, has high cholesterol and high blood pressure. He will pay $60.30 per month. That's $27.90 more per month than his healthy brother!

Over the 10 year period, the unhealthy brother will pay $3,348.00 more–that is just on premiums for being unhealthy! That is not even factoring in the amount of money spent on a 10 year period of monthly bills for cholesterol and high blood pressure medications.

**If you are 60 years old, then you will pay even more.**

A healthy female age 60 will pay $161 a month for $500,000 10 Year Term insurance.

An unhealthy female age 60 will pay $317 a month for $500,000 10 Year Term insurance. That is a difference of $18,720.00 difference over 10 years!

---

NOTE: You are deemed unhealthy by insurance companies if you have any of the following: high blood pressure, high cholesterol, or obesity.

Isn't that crazy?! So just looking at those statistics from the chiropractic wellness study above, along with the staggering difference in insurance premiums, doesn't it make financial sense take care of yourself and invest in your health right now?

## IT'S ALL ON WHAT YOU VALUE

The other day I met a man who said that he couldn't afford chiropractic care. That same man, I saw in the grocery store buying organic red peppers and cigarettes! It wasn't that he couldn't afford it; it was just that he didn't value it enough to want to truly change his life, and commit to taking care of himself. There is a difference. If you value something and want to make a change, you will do whatever it takes, even if it requires some temporary sacrifices.

I can tell you that chiropractors make their fees affordable (and many have affordable family plans), so that the entire family can receive chiropractic care. If a person truly values chiropractic care and is ready to make a commitment to their health, we are happy to work with them and find a way.

> **The Price of Crisis**
> Let me tell you firsthand about why I think Chiropractic care is ridiculously inexpensive in comparison to the amount spent on crisis care as a result of poor lifestyle choices.
>
> In January 2014, my dad was playing hockey and he suddenly collapsed in the center of the rink. He was having a heart attack!
>
> Fortunately, he survived, thanks to his teammates who took immediate action and used a portable defibrillator to save his life.
>
> In general, my Dad has been fit all his life, and he eats a fairly healthy diet. He had a history of smoking for 20 years and quit in his mid fifties. He saw his local

chiropractor 'once in a while', but was not motivated to go on a weekly or bi-monthly basis. Nor did he not want to do the initial work on correcting his rounded shoulder posture or spine to improve his overall nervous system function.

Thank God he survived the heart attack; however, shortly after, it was discovered that he needed a triple bypass surgery, due to clogged arteries and an electrical problem in the cardiac conduction system. Fortunately, his surgery was a success and he is doing well now. In terms of expenses incurred from this crisis, under Canadian health care, you might consider this "free" care. And yes, you don't have to pay a dime. But here's what you do have to pay for: Medications, a special chair to accommodate standing to sitting transitions, a commode, time off work for yourself, in addition to the costs incurred from those who are taking time off work to tend to you. What about your new travel insurance rates now? And ongoing medications? Or extra nursing care assistance? By the way, a Hyper-kyphotic thoracic spine, meaning rounded shoulders, is associated with an increased mortality rate.[81] Hmmm…. It doesn't look like corrective chiropractic care is too expensive now, does it?

Wouldn't it make sense to invest in your health now while it truly is affordable, so that you are functioning at your best healthy version of you?

# WHY DOESN'T MY MD REFER ME TO A CHIROPRACTOR?

*"Look to the spine for the cause of disease."*
*~Hippocrates-Father of Modern Medicine*

Most medical doctors are simply not aware of how chiropractic care can help their patients improve their overall health. If your medical doctor objects to you seeing a chiropractor, I suggest you ask them why. And follow up with "What research do you have to support this?" The opinions that we formulate, as professionals or parents, might not be as reliable if they are based on one singular experience. In my opinion, it is best to do your own research, get second opinions, and then make your own decisions that line up with your family values.

Medical doctors are trained on crisis care and are excellent at trauma care. Their focus is mainly for symptom based disease care. Chiropractors are focused on the cause of the problem and look to the spine for the cause of dis-ease.

A medical doctor (MD) and a chiropractor (DC), while different, have both received a degree from a government accredited medical school or Chiropractic College and are licensed to practice. But that's where the similarity ends because each discipline looks at health and healing in very different ways.

| Medical Doctors | Chiropractors |
| --- | --- |
| •Sees the disease | •Sees the person with the disease |
| •Relies on drugs | •Reduces causes of nerve interference |
| •Treats symptoms | •Promotes proper bodily function |

Clearly, these are two very different philosophies. Yet, each has its place. If you have broken bones or you're bleeding by the side of the road, you want the heroic lifesaving measures of emergency medical treatment. But if you have chronic aches and pains or an interest in wellness, you may want to choose a better way— Chiropractic.

## CAN CHIROPRACTIC HELP WITH PREGNANCY?

Yes, it can. Chiropractic care for the pregnant woman helps to keep the pelvis in proper alignment to allow optimum room for the baby to grow and move. It also helps alleviate nagging low back pain that many pregnant women report.

Studies have shown that over 50% of pregnant women experience low back pain and or sacroiliac pain during pregnancy.[82] Women who received chiropractic care showed a 95% improvement in their symptoms, in as little as 2 visits. [83] Research has shown that Chiropractic care shortened labor by as much as 31%. [84] Lastly, post partum depression was found to be rare in women who were under chiropractic care.[85]

The International Chiropractic Pediatric Association explains how beneficial chiropractic is:

In the Mother, Chiropractic:

- Relaxes the muscles and ligaments of the mother's pelvis.
- Restores neural integrity to the mother's uterus and cervix.
- Prepares the pelvis for easier delivery reducing unfavorable effects on the woman's pelvis.

To the infant:

- Allows the baby the room to resume proper position in-utero removing undue stress to the fetus' spine because of malposition.
- With proper fetal positioning, there is a significant decrease in birth trauma caused by intervention.

123

Many birth traumas can be a result of a malposition of the baby in the women's body. At 38 weeks, if the baby's head is not pointing down, the baby will be termed 'breech'. In this case we use a simple and gentle chiropractic technique called the 'Webster Technique". Along with thousands of other chiropractors, I am a certified expert in the Webster In-Utero Constraint technique, which "is a specific chiropractic analysis and adjustment used to correct misalignments in the mother's sacrum and pelvis. This relaxes the mother's pelvic muscles and ligaments, providing the physiological environment necessary for normal baby positioning." Doctors of Chiropractic reported an >85% success rate in its ability to balance pelvic structures and remove constraint to the woman's uterus therefore allowing the baby to turn into the proper head down position.[86]

## MY MIDWIFE SUGGESTED I SEE A CHIROPRACTOR. IS IT SAFE?

Yes, it is. First of all, the growing fetus is enveloped in amniotic fluid, which completely protects the baby growing inside the uterus, so a chiropractic adjustment cannot physically hurt the fetus.

Secondly, many chiropractors have adjusting tables that have special modifications to accommodate the pregnancy figure. In our center, along with many family chiropractic centers, we also have pregnancy pillows, which have a carved depression specifically to allow the mother to comfortably lie on her stomach while receiving her adjustment. In fact, many of our pregnant patients ask to borrow our pregnancy pillows because they are so comfortable for them. As the expectant mother is growing, adaptive techniques are used to adjust the mother's spine.

I always recommend choosing a Midwife for your pregnancy and birth. Chiropractors and midwives share a common objective and that is to eliminate as many variables that lead to traumatic birth, and create a healthy state for balance pre and post birth. Dr. Jeanie Om, Director of the International Chiropractic Pediatric Association, states "Midwives are referring patients to chiropractors even before mal-presentations are evident; and their practices are reaping the benefits of easier, safer deliveries for both mother and baby."

For both of my pregnancies, I had two fabulous midwives. Both times, they attended our at-home water birth and the pre and postnatal care and the care we received was exceptional! My daughter's birth was 8 hours and my son's birth was 4 hours. Both children were born safely at home in a water birthing pool. I attribute their smooth and easy birth to the regular chiropractic care and Midwifery care I received.

## WHY DO KIDS NEED CHIROPRACTIC?

Children need chiropractic for all different reasons. In fact there can be any number of stressors that may cause misalignments in your child's spine.

Probably the most common amongst these is childbirth. If you have had the privilege of being present at a birth you will understand why. Birth can involve quite a lot of force going through a baby's spine and nervous system – especially in the modern world, where the rates of hospital interventions like vacuum and caesarean sections are so high. In fact these stressors are so strong that it has been suggested that the first spinal problems experienced by over 80% of people actually began at birth.[87][88]

Did you know that 65% of neurological development

occurs in your child's first year? [89]

As we know, kids do lots of other stuff too. Whether it is the bumps and falls of learning to walk, sitting slumped over a desk all day at school, sports injuries, carrying heavy backpacks (over one shoulder) or learning to ride a bike, kids do stuff every day that has the potential to cause subluxations in their spine.

It makes sense to check kids for subluxations so that they can maximize their nerve function during these critical periods in their development and prevent problems that could potentially become much bigger problems later in life.[90]

*"When my daughter, Maya, first came to New Hope Chiropractic, she had quite a few challenges such as attention problems, immune problems, and constant emotional outbursts. Maya had a challenging firth and had gotten stuck at the neck and shoulders. After seeing Dr. Ron and Dr. Jody, we found out that Maya had quite a few challenges in her posture. Particularly in the upper part of her neck. We have been coming for 6 months and within that short time, she had completely changed. Her x-ray at 6 months had shown that her spine was completely restored back to a normal healthy curve! Her teachers all mentioned a noted improvement in Maya's attention and cooperation at school. Her immune system is 80% better than last year. I am so grateful to Dr. Jody and Dr. Ron for restoring health back to my family. It has truly changed her life!"*

*-Tanya*

# HOW DO I KNOW IF MY CHILD HAS A SUBLUXATION?

The short answer is, you may not. Kids can have subluxations and nerve interference long before they have any noticeable symptoms, but there may be a few obvious signs. If your child has disturbed sleeping patterns, if they have difficulty breast-feeding and attaching, if they have restricted neck movement or if they have one shoulder higher than the other then it is worthwhile getting a check-up from a Chiropractor.

If your child is displaying symptoms like recurrent ear infections, repeated sore throats, asthma, scoliosis, headaches, bedwetting, constipation or ADHD it may be a good idea to get a check-up. The aim of chiropractic care is not to treat any of these conditions (or any other symptoms), but merely to remove any interference and allow the body to adapt, repair and regenerate itself. As a result, parents and children will often notice an improvement in their symptoms too. What's even more exciting is that studies have shown that Chiropractic children are generally healthier than non-chiropractic children. [91] Specifically, a study showed a lower antibiotic use and a lower incidence of disease.[92]

Another study reported that 69% of the chiropractic children (kids who receive regular chiropractic care) have never had an ear infection.[93]

It goes back to the main principle of Vitalistic Model of Health Care, which is that your body knows how to heal itself. Chiropractic helps to improve that healing capability.

# DO CHIROPRACTORS USE THE SAME TYPE OF ADJUSTMENTS ON A CHILD AS AN ADULT? WILL IT HURT THEM?

No, chiropractic adjustments do not hurt a child (nor adults for that matter). Techniques used on children and babies are modified (more gentle) but the principle is exactly the same. In fact, many children love being adjusted because feels so good. The concern that many parents have is that chiropractic adjustments will be too forceful. They mistakenly think that their child will receive adjustments like ones they receive. The amount of pressure used to adjust a small baby would be about the amount of pressure you could comfortably apply to your eyeball without it hurting. In other words, not much! Because children are so flexible and don't have the years of built up spinal damage like adults often do, they respond brilliantly to chiropractic care. Typically chiropractors and parents see changes in kids' health and well-being much quicker than in adults.

# WHY WOULD A CHILD HAVE A SPINAL PROBLEM?

Traumatic births. Learning to walk. Slips. Falls. The list is endless. Yet, because children have such an adaptive capacity, these problems are often brushed off as "growing pains" or just a "phase they're going through." That is simply not the truth. As cited in Dr. Jennifer Barham-Floreani's book, Well-Adjusted Babies, research shows that on average, by the time a child turns the age of seven, they will have fallen over 2,500 times. Before the age of three, will have had three major falls off change tables, off a bed or down a flight of stairs. It is estimated that 47.9% of children land on their head in their first year of life.[94]

These 'micro' (small) or 'macro' (big) traumas over time can alter the developing structure of the body, and later on manifest as a symptom or dis-ease for the child.[95]

Many parents report that chiropractic care has been helpful for colic, ear infections, erratic sleeping habits, bedwetting, scoliosis, and many other common childhood health complaints. For example, a study showed that 94% of colic cases improved through chiropractic care.[96] Another study regarding ear infections showed 93% of all episodes improved, 75% in

10 days or fewer, and 43% with only one or two chiropractic adjustments.[97]

Parents with children under chiropractic care see an almost instant improvement in the well-being of their child.

We hear endless reports from parents that their children have not needed antibiotics, or that their child's behavior has improved since having chiropractic care.

Did you know that kids who are under chiropractic care also perform better academically? Yes, because not only is their nervous system and brain function improving, but also because they can sit longer in chairs without feeling aches or pains from chronic spinal misalignment and therefore can focus their attention longer on their school work.

Both our children, now aged 8 and 10, were checked for subluxations and adjusted within minutes of being born. They have since received regular chiropractic adjustments and we can attest that both children have never received an antibiotic nor drug for anything. Not only that, every single teacher they have had reports that they are incredible students, well behaved and have great physical abilities, including agility and balance. Our kids are far from perfect, and yes they get the odd cold but they recover within a day or two. Our kids can test our parental limits just like any other child. But there is no question that their nervous systems are functioning at a higher capacity with regular chiropractic adjustments, which gives them a better opportunity to be healthier all around.

## EVEN IF MY CHILD DOESN'T HAVE ANY PROBLEMS, SHOULD I STILL BRING THEM TO A CHIROPRACTOR?

Yes. Many young children will not be able to communicate to the parent that they have something wrong, but they may show signs of subluxation manifesting in other ways. For example, when newborns develop a bald spot on the back of their head, it is typically a result of a subluxation in their upper spine and the baby is innately trying to correct it by rotating their head back and forth, thus continually rubbing the back of their head resulting in a 'bald spot'.

Another simple way to tell if your baby has a possible subluxaton, is if they are not breastfeeding on both sides equally. If a newborn is struggling to fully attach onto the nipple, it may be due to the infant's inability to properly open their jaw, which may be due to a misalignment in the jaw joint or upper neck. If your baby is colicky, it may be a sign of nerve interference, and chiropractic can help.

Even if your child doesn't have any symptoms of dis-ease, you really can't tell if they have a subluxation unless checked by a chiropractor. Just like you can't tell if your child has a dental cavity, you really can't tell if they have a subluxation in their spine. In a way, chiropractic is just like the dentist, but for your spine and nervous system. Remember, that chiropractic reduces subluxation and restores and maintains proper alignment within the spine.

*"As the twig is bent, so grows the tree."*
*-Chinese proverb*

*I have always been a firm believer in Chiropractic care, so when I became pregnant with twins, I continued with my treatments, and my body was able to successfully carry them to full term. Once the girls were born and were a few weeks old, I introduced them to Dr. Jody and their journey began. One of my daughters, Madeline, had a flat back of the head, and it appeared from the very beginning that her neck or back was uncomfortable as she wiggled and moved her body while crying and fussing. As a mother I was deeply concerned about our newborn and Dr. Jody assured me she would be able to help. Within a few weeks of extremely gentle massage and manipulation it became obvious that she was feeling better. As we have continued with her adjustments over the years she is a happy, comfortable 5 year old who receives an adjustment every few weeks to keep her growing in alignment. Madeline's sister and brother also enjoy Chiropractic Care as a part of their healthy upbringing. It has been proven to our family that when our bodies and spines are aligned properly, not only do we grow healthy and strong but we also have fewer colds and flus than many of our peers. Our family views our Chiropractors as experts in our body's physical functions, and we feel that giving our children the gift of Chiropractic care sets them up for a lifetime of success.*

*-Sabrina V.*

# WHAT SHOULD I DO IN CRISIS?

The first thing I always tell our babysitter is that if there is an emergency, "Take action with wise eyes." Our kids have fortunately never been to a hospital for crisis yet. There was a time when our daughter split the back of her head open when she was 4 years old. There was so much blood and the gap was too big to leave it. I hauled her into the walk-in clinic and met with our Family "Emergency/Crisis" doctor. We call them Emergency/Crisis Doctors only because that is when we would need to use their services and expertise — in emergency and crisis.

After assessing the situation for our daughter, our Emergency/Crisis Doctor decided that she was going to need several stitches. At the time of the event, it was in the middle of a Norwalk virus outbreak at our only hospital where we were supposed to go get the stitches. I challenged our Emergency/Crisis Doctor to come up with an alternative plan, and after some creative brainstorming, a solution was met. It was decided that after the wound was cleaned, we would braid her hair tightly to close over the wound. This would bring the edges together like stitches, and then we would seal the wound by applying a Bitumen Balm creating a waterproof anti-infection seal. Does this sound crazy? Nope. This technique has been utilized for thousands of years in many places across the globe.

So we saved our little girl from needing a local anesthetic injection and subjecting her to potential endless hours waiting in the hospital—all through using "Wise Eyes". Years later, we still enjoy this story as it goes to show that even in the medical profession, there are some natural alternatives that are very effective. You just have to ask.

When it comes to crisis, our family plan is as follows: discern the situation, take appropriate action with wise eyes, and give assurance and love.

People often ask me about what to do when they have a fall or injure themselves, should they apply heat or cold. In acute (meaning, sudden) instances, we stick to the well-known "RICE" protocol:

**R**est

**I**ce

**C**ompress

**E**levate.

This is for simple injuries such as a muscle strain. If you feel it is more serious, definitely seek Emergency/Crisis Medical care.

## COLD THERAPY

When it comes to ice therapy, I suggest the CBAN method: Apply a cold compress over the injured area (not directly on the skin), and then time your treatment according to what you experience in the following steps:

Cold: you will first feel a cold sensation

Burning sensation — keep going

Aching —keep going and finally it will feel Numb.

When you feel a numbing sensation on the area, then you can stop the therapy. It should take approximately 20 minutes. Do not let your ice therapy go beyond the 20 minutes. If you do exceed that time frame, your intelligent body will start to think that something is wrong with this cold bodily area. As a result it will start a process to try and warm it up, hence creating the opposite effect of what you are trying to achieve.

## HOMEOPATHIC THERAPY

Homeopathic medicine is effectively used to stimulate the body's own healing response to a disease using diluted and prepared natural resources, typically in the form of a plant or mineral. They come in tiny pellet forms and you can pick them up at health food stores. We have four general homeopathic medicines that we have on hand for trauma or crisis. If you have more specific health concerns, you should consult a professional homeopath. I always refer my patients to a homeopath when they want to reduce or eliminate a medication. I have seen first-hand patients who have committed to making changes in their lifestyle, including getting chiropractic care, and the help of a homeopath, successfully stop taking a lifetime of drugs. Here are the ones that are great to have in your first aid kit:

**Belladonna**: use for sudden high fever. Usually the person is red and flushed with dilated pupils.

**Arnica**: excellent for the pain, shock, swelling and bleeding of any injury. It can be taken immediately and frequently, as the pain subsides, take it less frequently.

**Traumeel**: great for acute pain and you can put it like an ointment on sprained ankles or bruised muscles. Also we have traumeel eardrops, which come in handy for sudden acute ear pain or cabin pressure changes during an airplane flight.

**Oculoheel eye drops**: is a homeopathic preparation to relieve minor conjunctivitis, inflammation, irritation, burning sensation, watery eyes, itching, and redness.

# WHAT CAN CHIROPRACTIC DO FOR ME?

By now, you are probably aware of the amazing power inside you, the health model options available, and how having a healthy spine and nervous system allows you do to enjoy a better life. But you still might be wondering specifically how chiropractic can help you.

Understand that chiropractic can help with *everything*— why, because removing interference in your nervous system improves the function of your nervous system, including brain function.[98] And if your nervous system is functioning at a higher level, then guess what?- everything that the nervous system controls should also be functioning at a higher level.

While many chiropractic studies point to the obvious low back pain benefits and preventing surgeries[99], many studies now show the benefits of overall health, including boosting immunity and enhancing DNA repair.[100] For example: Chiropractic patients had a 200% greater immune- competence than people who had no chiropractic care. [101] DNA repair (your body's building blocks) was reported to be most effective in individuals who had been receiving long term chiropractic care. [102] Chiropractic adjustments have been shown to significantly lower blood pressure. [103] [104] And even studies have shown a reduction in stress hormones following chiropractic adjustments. [105] How awesome is that?!

Even athletes benefit from chiropractic care as they experience that their bodies work more efficiently so they can get better performance with no increase in effort. In a study showing chiropractic's effectiveness, competitive cyclists (4 men and 2 women) were able to measurably improve their performance after just one to two weeks of chiropractic care.[106]

*Now where to begin....as far back as Grade 8, I've been in a lot of pain. I was told by a number of people, and three different doctors, that I had fibromyalgia. At the end of high school, I was in so much pain, that I would punch myself in the head to ease the pain. It felt as if I had sand in my veins. A year later, I had a brain hemorrhage. Still in pain, I was suffering now with seizures, and forced to be on welfare, and now on permanent disability. Then one day, just a couple weeks ago, I saw a chiropractor for the first time. I have been without pain for two weeks straight since starting chiropractic care 3 weeks ago. My neck doesn't need to be massaged every night anymore. I am standing straight, and feeling great, for the first time in my life. I've told everyone, who knows what I've been through, about the amazing changes I have experienced through chiropractic care at New Hope Chiropractic. I feel like I have been given my life back! Thank You.*

*- Steven H.*

## CAN CHIROPRACTIC HELP ME GET OFF MY MEDICATIONS?

Your body is designed to be healthy. It is not deficient of drugs or medications. We will never tell you to stop your medication, but we will direct you in the proper steps on how you can begin changes. Having said that, research shows that chiropractic patients demonstrated 85% less pharmaceutical costs when compared with patients under conventional medicine. [107]

# HOW ABOUT ASTHMA? ALLERGIES? STOMACH PAIN? OR (FILL IN THE BLANK)?

Chiropractic care has shown time and time again that by removing the interference in the spine you are allowing the body to heal itself the way it is supposed to.

Experts agree that reducing exposure to pollution, eating "clean", moving your body, all help with keeping the body healthy, but chiropractic care has also been shown to reduce symptoms in both kids and adults alike. Why? Because another significant reason that contributes to the onset of asthma, or even digestive issues[108] has to do with poor spinal health.

Patients under regular chiropractic care have enhanced nerve system function and therefore have better immune competence and a greater capacity to resist disease[109]

> *"I grew up with chronic asthma and dealt with it for all of my adult life. I was addicted to inhalers and never thought that I would be free of them. After doing much spiritual work and healing the core issues of my illness through chiropractic, I am happy to say that I am asthma free! I have been under chiropractic care for over three years and have been able to stop all medication. My immune system is healed, my spirit restored and life is beautiful!"*

> *-Lori P.*

Chiropractic doesn't treat any ailments or symptoms, because when a chiropractic adjustment restores the nerve distortion, then your body naturally responds and begins the healing cascade, ultimately restoring things back to normal. To learn more about the positive effects of chiropractic and gain access to research on a variety of health related topics, then please visit: www.icpa4kids.org and click on Chiropractic Research.

## HOW CAN I CONVINCE MY SPOUSE TO GET CHIROPRACTIC CARE?

First tip: Don't nag.

Just like trying to convince someone to quit smoking because you know they will have a healthier life if they quit, nagging techniques do not work. Motivation to see a chiropractor comes from either pain or motivation to become healthier.

Encouragement and acceptance are best. And typically, as your spouse sees improvement in your health and vitality, chances are they will be more attracted to it for themselves. So leading by example is always best. In our office, we encourage couples to come together, so they can support each other through the process of restoration, and move towards higher levels of health and vitality as a couple and or family.

Second tip: Start with a check-up, not care. You are not convincing them to commit to chiropractic care. They are just taking the next step, and that is a chiropractic consultation and exam. Without getting complicated and trying to figure it all out. Keep it simple, and start with taking the next step. Start with a chiropractic check-up, first. That's it.

# PART FOUR:

## Life Giving Recipes

There are so many amazing blog recipe sites where you can look up just about any type of recipe you want, and I have referenced some of my favorite websites at the end of this book. However, these particular recipes are my 'Tried and True' Go To's. Every single recipe is designed to nourish your body and each ingredient has a healthy life giving purpose. Not only that, they are easy to assemble in advance which cuts down in prep time in the kitchen. Anyone can make them -whether it is a two year old who can add vegetable toppings onto his plate to create a taco salad, or the grandfather who is learning how to make a simple yet, powerfullyhealthy, smoothie.

Lastly, 96% of everything we eat is life giving (or 'Vision food'). When you know you are having something that is good for you, you will enjoy it that much more

For more recipes that we continually test and update into our family meals visit: www.drjodycox.com.

# Healing Drinks

## ARISE AND FLUSH DRINK

This lemon drink creates an instant detox and helps to flush out toxins in your body. We have this drink every single day, first thing in the morning. Wait for at least 30 minutes before you consume anything else so that you reap the health benefits of establishing a good alkaline base in your body to start your day. One mistake I hear about people who try this drink, is that they use cold water. Cold water first thing in the morning can totally shock your system, whereas using warm water (or body temperature water) is much better for the first drink of your day. I also recommend using fresh lemons as opposed to buying the liquid lemon. I know it is more work, but it is totally worth it to have a fresh enzyme release of pure lemon into your body.

*Ingredients*

2-3 cups warm or hot water

½ lemon squeezed

## UPGRADED MORNING DRINK

We make this drink at night, let it sit and enjoy it first thing in the morning. We add 1 tsp of baking soda to the lemon water drink. This furthers an alkaline environment in the body and the combination has anti-carcinogenic properties.

# TURMERIC, HONEY & GINGER TEA

This is a warm and cozy drink, great for the evening after dinner or on a chilly weekend morning. Turmeric and Ginger combined are anti-inflammatory and help ease bloating. You can use almond milk, or open a can of coconut milk. I pre-mix equal portions of the spices together and store in a small mason jar so that it is ready to go.

*Ingredients*

>   1 cup water
>
>   ¼ teaspoon ground turmeric
>
>   ¼ teaspoon ground ginger
>
>   Splash of almond milk
>
>   Raw honey, to taste

*Directions*

Add turmeric and ginger into a mug. Fill with boiling water, let sit for a few minutes.

Stir in almond milk. Add honey and enjoy! Serves 1.


# GREEN TEA

We drink green tea regularly in our household. It is so tasty and known for its antioxidant properties. It is also known to help keep unwanted pounds off your body.

# Smoothies

Our family enjoys smoothies a few times a week. I typically make a smoothie for more of an afterschool meal for my kids when they are in transition from school to sports activities. This is a great way to fuel up on some healthy fats and replenish their caloric needs, while enjoying a nurturing yummy drink. This has been a routine in our family for years and I love that it is so easy to make, clean up, and enjoy in such a short time. For those of you who have picky eaters, now is your chance to throw in those avocados, or hemp hearts, or nuts, or kale, that your little one might not necessarily want to eat at that time ;). If you are looking to add more protein to your meal, you can add 1-2 pastured eggs (raw, local, organic) to your smoothies.


Note: all smoothie recipes make enough for about 1 liter – approximately 2+ servings.

# GREEN GLORY SMOOTHIE

This is the smoothie that we make most often as it is loaded with those highly nutritious, antioxidant dark leafy greens. We use it to offset a day or week that we might not have consumed as many greens as we were hoping to. And rather than battle it out the odd time with my kids to eat their greens, I am happy to use this graciously!

## *Ingredients*

   1 banana

   ½ avocado

   1 Tbsp. almond or hazelnut butter

   1 cup frozen berries

   2 cups organic spinach, kale or swiss chard

   2 cups water, coconut water, or unsweetened almond milk

   1 tsp cinnamon

## *Directions*

Blend in high-speed blender until smooth.

# DATE SMOOTHIE

Dates are a good source of fiber and contain high levels of the essential minerals potassium, magnesium, copper, and manganese. We only use Medjool dates because they are superior in size and texture. Serves 2 +

## *Ingredients*

   3 medjool dates

   ½ banana

   ½ c macadamia nuts

   2 cups unsweetened almond milk

   1 Tbsp. coconut oil (extra virgin)

   1 tbsp. pure vanilla extract or vanilla powder

   Ice (optional)

## *Directions*

Blend away until color is a latte color. Enjoy!

# STRAWBERRY DREAMS SMOOTHIE

Strawberries are a great source of Vitamin C and Hemp Hearts are a powerful source of protein. You will love the color of this smoothie.

## *Ingredients*

>   5-6 frozen strawberries 2 Tbsp. hemp hearts
>
>   ¼ lemon (with rind)
>
>   2 cups water or coconut water
>
>   ½ banana
>
>   ½ avocado

## *Directions*

Blend until lemon rind is no longer in bits, but smoothed into the drink.

# BLUEBERRY FIELDS SMOOTHIE

These low sugar berries are rated as the highest in antioxidant activity when compared to 40 other fresh fruits and vegetables. They are known for their protection against cancer and heart disease. Aside from that, blueberries are our favorite fruit, and we go to great lengths to pick up boxes of them every summer and freeze them so we can continue to enjoy them throughout the winter. Serves 2

### Ingredients

> 1 cup frozen blueberries
>
> 1 cup frozen cranberries
>
> 1 tbsp almond butter
>
> 2-3 cups coconut water
>
> ½ avocado
>
> tbsp Holy Crap cereal
>
> 2 dates

### Directions

Blend on high for 2 minutes.

# Fresh Juices

Fresh juices provide a massive dose of nutrition that is very easy for your body to absorb. Your body gets deep nourishment and hydration, while the digestive system gets a break from processing the heavier foods we normally eat. We have an Omega Vert Juicer and we love it. It's easy to clean, easy to assemble and it's very powerful. There are plenty of varieties of juices (just experiment!), but here are the two main ones we make on a regular basis. Juicing is a good idea when you need a 'detox' or your digestive system needs a well-deserved break, or you are recovering from an illness. Serves 2+

## GOOD MORNING JUICE

*Ingredients*

 2 handfuls of spinach

 2 handfuls of kale

 Half a bunch of cilantro and parsley (each)

 2 apples, cored

 2 lemons, peeled and cut

 A knob of peeled fresh ginger

 1 medium cucumber, sliced

 2 stalks of celery

# KID'S FAVORITE JUICE

*Ingredients*

5 carrots

3 apples

3 celery stalks

1 beet (optional)

# Breakfasts

Breakfasts are a big deal in our home and should be in yours too. Don't skip it, or minimize it. It will set your day and body's metabolism in the right direction.


## JULIA CHILD OMELET

I taught my kids to make omelets when they were young so that they would have a skill in the kitchen when it comes to a healthy protein source that is easy to make. We loved watching Julia Child's old TV series, The French Chef. Since then, my kids are professional omelet makers! It takes literally 5 minutes and clean up is quicker than any other breakfast concoction. Serves 1.

*Ingredients*

2 farm fresh eggs

Salt and pepper

1 tbsp of Organic butter, coconut oil or Ghee

*Directions*

Melt 1 tbsp of fat in a frying pan on high heat. Whip up two eggs in a small bowl and add salt and pepper. Once the butter is almost golden, slide in the blended eggs. Count to 10 and then shuffle your pan vigorously back and forth for at least 2 minutes, until the omelet is just solid. Then slide the omelet from the pan directly onto a plate and turn the pan as to fold over the omelet. Bon Appetit!

# BREAKFAST BOWL

This is a nice hearty meal that comes in handy on chilly winter mornings, or provides a great comfort meal. You can typically ground the walnut and almonds days before and store in a jar for up to 2 weeks. That way, your mix is ready to go in the morning.

## *Ingredients*

> 1 cup Gluten Free oats, or 1 cup ground Walnut and Almonds
>
> 2 organic eggs
>
> ½ mashed banana
>
> 1 cup unsweetened almond milk or coconut milk
>
> ¼ cup large unsweetened flaked coconut
>
> ¼ cup pumpkin seeds
>
> 2 tbsp of hemp hearts and chia seeds (each) or 2 tbsp of Holy Crap cereal
>
> 2 tbsp cinnamon
>
> Frozen blueberries

## *Directions*

Mix together the eggs, add mashed banana and milk. Then add the oats or nut mix and cook on medium in a saucepan for 20 minutes. Once the mixture is fully cooked, stir in all of the remaining ingredients. Place on top of a bowl or jar lined with blueberries. Serves 2+ (Adapted from Dr. David Perlmutter's book, Grain Brain.)

# SALMON PANCAKES

Yes, salmon pancakes are one of our favorite easy peasy breakfasts and loaded with protein and omega 3 nutrients! Makes 20+ small pancakes.

## *Ingredients*

1 can of wild pacific canned salmon

2 eggs

2 Tbsps. almond meal (ground almonds)

2 Tbsp. minced shallot or onion

2 tsp. Holy Crap cereal

Pepper

## *Directions*

Mix all ingredients together in a bowl. Heat a frying pan with Ghee or coconut oil. Scoop 1/4 cup of mix into pan and fry as you would a pancake. Turn over and continue (about 3 minutes per side). Serve with salsa or chutney.

# 2 INGREDIENT PROTEIN PANCAKES

When I was a student and didn't have much time or money to make or create meals, this recipe was a miracle. Funny enough, 25 years later, this recipe continues to be a hit in our family. Quick to make, and most likely gobbled up before it hits the plate. Did I mention it is highly nutritious and has 12 grams of protein?? Serves 1+

### *Ingredients*

> 1 egg
>
> 1 soft banana

### *Directions*

Mash the banana in a small bowl till almost pureed. Beat in the egg. Melt 1 tbsp of coconut oil in a frying pan over medium low heat. Pour approx. ¼ cup of batter to create your pancake. Gently flip in 3 minutes (watch for small bubbles). No need to add anything, but you could top it off with almond butter, berries or cinnamon for a decadent rendition.

# EVERYDAY KETO PANCAKES

Keto refers to a fat burning diet that is low in carbs and high in quality fat. These pancakes are exactly that: fluffy, easy to make, and taste delicious. You can freeze these and toast them for later use.

## *Ingredients*

- 1 cup Almond flour
- ¼ cup Coconut flour
- 2 tbsp coconut sugar, or natural sweetener of your choice
- 1 tsp baking powder
- 6 large Eggs
- 6 tbsp Unsweetened almond milk (or any milk of choice)
- 1 tsp Vanilla
- 1 pinch Sea salt

## *Directions*

Whisk all ingredients together in a bowl until smooth. (Batter should be the consistency of typical pancake batter. If it's too thick, add a little more milk.)

Heat 2 tablespoons of grass fed-butter or coconut oil in a pan. Drop the batter onto the hot pan and form into circles. Cover and cook about 1.5-2 minutes, until bubbles start to form. Flip and cook another 1.5-2 minutes, until browned on the other side. Repeat with the rest of the batter.

# GRAIN FREE WEEKEND CEREAL

Yes, it does happen. Kids will eventually find out about that infamous cereal aisle. After all, it is the 'Vegas' of the grocery store. Bright colored boxes decorated with cartoon animals enticing kids with tricks and toys while deceptively promising Moms that the contents are truly healthy. I finally got sick and tired of 'interviewing' healthy cereals for approval for our home. It just wasn't worth my time searching for the holy grail of healthy cereals. So after lots of trial and error, I have finally mastered one that is grain free, refined sugar free, and packed with quality nutrients. Plus, the kids love it!!!


PS—Don't get discouraged about the long list of ingredients. Once you initially source the main ingredients, buy in bigger quantities. That way it will be easy to make regularly.

## Ingredients

- 2 cups sliced almonds
- 1 cup pumpkin seeds
- 1 cup sunflower seeds
- 1 cup unsweetened coconut flakes
- ½ cup hemp hearts
- ½ cup sesame seeds
- ¼ cup chia seeds
- 4 medjool dates—pitted and chopped finely
- 1 handful of raisins
- ½ cup coconut oil
- ½ cup nut butter (almond or cashew is nice)
- ½ cup unsweetened applesauce
- 1 Tbsp cinnamon
- Tbsp vanilla

## Directions

Set oven to 375°F. Mix all flakes, hearts, cinnamon, nuts, and seeds (except Chia) in a large bowl.

Melt the coconut oil, nut butter, applesauce and vanilla in a small pan. Stir into the mix then pour into a large roasting pan. Bake for 15 minutes, stir in chopped dates, and bake again for 10 minutes. Once done, stir in raisins and chia seeds. Cool and store in large glass jars for 2 weeks (if it lasts that long). Serve with your favorite milk or Kefir.

# Spice Mixes and Dressings

Two time saver spices that I pre-mix about once a month are the Warming Spice Mix and Taco Mix. I just don't like to get into the middle of a recipe and then find myself climbing through my spices and measuring—it is just too much of a fuss for me. So I make these two highly utilized spice mixes and store them in our cabinet. We use them in so many dishes— from tacos, to soups, or pancakes, oatmeal, or even in a tea. Just get two recycled jam jars, pull out your spices and make these as you will most likely appreciate the easy access to them anytime.

The dressings are all amazing and very versatile and you can interchange them with most salads and bowls.

# NATURAL TACO MIX

You can always buy an organic taco mix in the store, but making your own will save you money and you can monitor the salt ingredients. I make the spice in bulk, and store it in a mason jar so that it is easily ready for use. You can also add a few teaspoons of it to a soup for added flavor.

## *Ingredients*

½ cup chili powder

2 ½ teaspoons garlic powder

2 ½ teaspoons onion powder

2 ½ teaspoons red pepper flakes

2 ½ teaspoons oregano

2 ½ teaspoons paprika

¼ cup plus 1 tablespoon cumin

¼ cup Himalayan salt (more to taste)

¼ cup finely ground pepper

## *Directions*

Combine in Mason jar, label and store in cupboard.

# COMFORT SPICE MIX

This spice mix was passed down to me from my Mom. It can be used on any roasted root vegetable, soups, baked apples or added to a beef stew for extraordinary flavor.

## *Ingredients*

1 Tbsp ground ginger

2 Tbsp cinnamon

½ tsp cloves

½ tsp nutmeg

½ tsp allspice

## *Directions*

Combine in small jam jar and store in cupboard.

# PUMPKIN GINGER DRESSING

This is a quick dressing that you can pretty much put on any veggie bowl, or use as a salad dressing, veggie dip, or a spread in your wraps. I recently put it onto a plate of steamed asparagus, tuna and a plate of rice noodles— turned out fabulous! Adapted from blogger Sarah Britton of www.MyNewRoots.org.

*Ingredients*

¾ cup pumpkin seeds

¼ cup hemp hearts

3 cloves garlic

1 Tbsp fresh cut up ginger

1 Tbsp honey

3 Tbsp olive oil

1 Tbsp apple cider vinegar

3 Tbsp lemon juice

¾ - 1 cup water

salt and pepper

*Directions*

Blend all ingredients in a magic bullet or food processor. For dressing, add more water; for dip, add less. Store in a glass jar. Lasts in the fridge for 1 week.

# TAHINI MISO MAPLE DRESSING

Amazing on cold rice noodles, zucchini noodles, or with an assortment of vegetables.

## *Ingredients*

    ¼ c tahini

    2 tbsp miso paste

    1 tbsp maple syrup

    ¼ c water

## *Directions*

Blend all ingredients in a magic bullet or food processor. Store in a glass jar. Lasts in the fridge for 1 week.

# BASIC BALSAMIC DRESSING

Our go to dressing that is great on just about anything!

## *Ingredients*

> Juice from half a lime
>
> 2 tbsp tamari (it is a wheat-free version of soy sauce) or coconut aminos
>
> 2 tbsp maple syrup
>
> 4 Tbsp Balsamic Vinegar
>
> ¼ cup sesame oil or olive oil (extra virgin)
>
> 1 Tbsp Dijon mustard
>
> ¼ tsp. Himalayan or sea salt

## *Directions*

Blend and store in jam jar in fridge up to one week.

# HEMP CITRUS DRESSING

This is best on a coleslaw or chunky type of salad.

## *Ingredients*

 ¼ cup hemp hearts

 ¼ cup water

 2 medjool dates

 Juice from half a lemon

## *Directions*

Blend and store in jam jar in fridge up to one week.


# BASIC LEMON DRESSING

Great on sliced avocados or a bed or arugula .

Squeeze half lemon into 1/4 cup of olive oil, pinch of salt and pepper. Mix in a jam jar and store in fridge.

# "BEST EVER" CILANTRO PEANUT DRESSING

This is my favorite summer dressing and dip. Goes well on rice or kelp noodles, burgers, salads and steamed vegetables. Adapted from the kitchen of my talented friend, Stephanie Wiebe.

(ificouldiwould-stephanie.blogspot.com)

## *Ingredients*

3 whole big cloves of garlic

1 Tbsp fresh ginger

2 bunches cilantro, (rinsed well, most of stalk ends trimmed off)

½ cup fresh lime juice

1 ½ tsp wine vinegar/rice vinegar

1 tsp. ground cumin

¾ tsp. salt

½ tsp. freshly ground pepper

1 Tbsp. honey or 2 Medjool Dates

½ cup olive oil

4 Tbsp. almond butter

2 Tbsp. coconut aminos

## *Directions*

Put all the ingredients into food processor, except olive oil. Once everything is pureed and blended, slowly stream olive oil in so that the dressing becomes emulsified.

# Salads

These salads are quick and so filling. The bonus is that these salads will give you sustainable energy after lunch and avoid that heavy carbohydrate sluggish feeling.

## RAW ENERGY CHOP SALAD

A Quick refreshing lunch and the walnuts and seeds make it hearty. Serves 2+

*Ingredients*

> 2 apples
>
> 2 celery stalks Half a cucumber
>
> 2 cups chopped kale
>
> ½ cup walnuts
>
> Handful of pumpkin seeds

*Directions*

Chop all the fruit and vegetables and place into a bowl, toss in the walnuts, top with pumpkin seeds. Drizzle the Hemp Citrus Dressing on salad as you wish.

# VIBRANT SALAD

You will feel vibrant just looking at this salad. Serves 4

## *Ingredients*

2 ripe avocados - cut into chunks

½ head of romaine lettuce (8 leaves)—torn into small pieces

10-12 cherry tomatoes, cut in half

20 blanched green beans (cut)

Top with crushed nori seaweed, 1/4 cup pumpkin seeds and sunflower seeds

## *Directions*

Assemble all ingredients in a large bowl and toss with

Lemon Dressing.

Optional: you can toss in a chopped hard boiled egg and a can of ocean wise wild tuna or sardines; substitute the seaweed for 2 tablespoons of capers, and you have a healthy rendition of a Nicoise Salad.

# SPRING SALAD ROLLS or LAYERED SALAD

This is a stunning meal you can prepare in advance for dinner guests, or simply set up a 'creation station' for your family to add their own toppings.

At home, we layer the salad; but when we are picnicking, I take all the below ingredients and roll them up in a large rice paper wrap like a burrito.

Serves 6+ but you can adjust the ingredients to accommodate more or less.

*Ingredients*

1 Package of Brown rice vermicelli noodles, soaked in boiling water and drained.

1 bunch of spinach or romaine lettuce

4 Shredded carrots

1 Shredded cucumber

2 Green onions, sliced

2 Chopped avocadoes

½ Shredded purple cabbage

2 Red peppers, sliced

2 Mangoes, sliced

1 bunch of Cilantro

Optional: cooked chicken pieces, tuna, smoked salmon

*Directions*

Layer the above on top of a platter of rice noodles. Dressing or Dip (if making rolls) can be either any of the dressings above, but I particularly love the *Cilantro Peanut Dressing* with this.

# FRENCH POTATO SALAD SUPREME

A good friend of mine made this salad for me years ago, and since then I have made some adjustments. It is literally my 'go to' potluck salad that is pure delight.

## *Ingredients*

5 large white or red organic potatoes, cleaned, cubed.

½ large onion, diced

1 cup of Basic Balsamic Dressing

½ cup sundried tomatoes

¼ cup shredded parsley

## *Directions*

Steam potatoes for 15-20 minutes. Check for doneness. Gently drain and transfer to bowl. Once cooled, add the remainder of the ingredients and carefully fold in, so not to mash the potatoes. Enjoy! Serves 6.

# Bowls

These are a great way of enjoying a whole bunch of goodness packed into your own bowl. For the base of the bowl, use your favorite cooked noodle (brown vermicelli rice or buckwheat), rice, or quinoa. Then add your assortments of veggies and protein, and finally, top it off with a delicious dressing and crunch topping.

Sounds yummy? It is!

Don't want to use grains? Then simply make cauliflower rice, or zucchini noodles for the base.

# ABUNDANCE BOWL

## *Ingredients*

Base: (enough for 4 hungry people)

2 cups each of chopped kale and broccoli

1 cup of sun dried or cherry tomatoes

2 sweet potatoes

2 handfuls of sprouts of any kind

½ cup Sliced almonds

-For extra protein, add grilled fish or chicken.

## *Directions*

Cook noodles, quinoa or rice according to package. Drain, rinse cool, and place into bowls.

While your base is cooking, peel and thinly slice sweet potato. Place on a cookie sheet lined with parchment paper. Drizzle a spoonful of olive oil and set under the broiler for 4 minutes. Set aside.

Steam broccoli and kale for 4 minutes and set aside. Fill the bottom of each bowl with cooked base. Divide and add sweet potato, broccoli and kale. Add protein if using. Top with sun dried tomatoes, sprouts and almonds. Drizzle with dressing (Pumpkin Ginger or Basic Balsamic).

# QUICK POKE BOWL

Poke is the Hawaiian word for "to slice or cut". The key to making this fabulous dish is to have a very sharp knife. If you don't have tuna, you can use 4 cups of cooked shrimp or prawns. You can replace the rice with kelp noodles for a grain free meal. Serves 4+

## Ingredients

  4 Ahi Tuna filets

  1 avocado cut into small chunks

  ½ large cucumber diced

  12 cherry tomatoes cut in half

  1 mango cut into chunks

  4 cups cooked rice

  1 cup Gluten Free Teriyaki Sauce

  ½ cup finely chopped green onion

  2 tablespoons black sesame seed

## Directions

Place the ahi tuna into the freezer to chill for 15 minutes. Then with a sharp knife, cut tuna into half an inch strips and then cut on the perpendicular plane, so that you end up with small cubes of tuna. Do this for each fillet. Place tuna into a separate bowl and toss with the teriyaki sauce, green onion, and black sesame seeds.

Place equal portions of rice into 4 bowls. Arrange equal portions of the tuna on one side of each bowl on top of the rice.

Distribute the remaining ingredients equally alongside each other so that they are not mixed. Drizzle with extra sauce for added flavor.

# Soups

There are so many delicious soups out there, but our family's favorite soups are Zudon Noodle soup and Squash Soup. Both soup bases are so easy to make and can be repurposed in a variety of ways to create different meals. For example, you can take the squash soup, add a jar of salsa and cubed cooked chicken to make Mexican chicken chowder. The udon noodle soup broth can be recycled as a base for stir fry, or frozen into ice cube trays and then later used as a natural flavor enhancer to any soup, stew or poured over roasted vegetables. I typically will double the recipes when it comes to soup and then label and freeze in freezer bags for later use.

# ZUDON SOUP

My kids love udon noodle soup, but those thick white flour noodles are just not healthy.

Here is a much quicker and more nutritious noodle rendition using zucchini noodles instead. You need a spirolizer which you can pick up at any kitchen store to transform zuchinni into a noodle. You can always cut the zucchini into thin strips of noodles by hand—it just takes longer, but still works. Another option is to use soba buckwheat or brown rice noodles and cook according to package.

First create a soup base broth, create your zucchini noodles (or boil noodles, or brown rice noodles), and then you can add pretty much any chopped vegetable you like. Serves 4.

## *Ingredients*

Base broth:

8 cups of organic chicken broth.

¼ cup of Gluten Free Tamari or Coconut Aminos

1/8 cup of fish sauce (MSG free)

2 cloves of garlic, finely diced

1 tablespoon shredded ginger (or use 1 tsp. of powder ginger)

Dash of sesame oil

Heat up coconut oil in a soup pot and add garlic and ginger and sauté for a few minutes. Then add the remaining broth ingredients. Bring to a boil and then reduce heat to simmer.

## Zoodles:

While broth is heating, peel and slice 4 zucchinis and then use a julienne peeler, or spirolizer to create your noodles. You don't need to cook them because adding them to the hot broth will do the trick. If you are using brown rice noodles, or buckwheat noodles, first cook these according to package and drain and rinse in cold water. Divide the pile of noodles into four bowls.

**Veggies and Protein:**

Prepare an assortment of desired vegetables such as:

Thinly sliced carrots

Chopped broccoli Diced green onion

Chopped baby bok choy or napa cabbage. Chopped snap peas

Thinly sliced red pepper

Optional: chunks of pre-cooked chicken, or cooked shrimp.

*Directions*

Add the hearty vegetables such as broccoli, carrots and or cabbage into the boiling broth and let cook for three minutes. Next ladle your hot soup broth over each bowl of the noodles and vegetables until it covers all the ingredients in the bowl. Then cover the each bowl with a plate to lightly steam the veggies inside for 5 minutes. Remove the plate, put under your bowl and enjoy.

# COMFORT SQUASH SOUP

This is an easy and creamy comfort food that pleases just about anyone. Serves 4+

### Ingredients

1 large butternut squash, cut in half lengthwise and scoop out seeds

1 large onion, cut into quarters

5 carrots, cut in half

1 large yam or sweet potato, peeled and cubed

4 peeled and smashed garlic cloves

2 Tbsp coconut oil

8 cups of chicken broth

1 can full fat coconut milk

1 Tbsp Comfort Spice Mix

### Directions

Heat oven to 350°F. Place all vegetables in a large roasting pan. Add the coconut oil—if it is firm, don't worry, it will melt itself into the vegetables later on. Cover pan with tin foil and bake for 40 minutes. Once cool, scoop out squash from its skin and put all vegetables into a large pot. Puree the vegetables with an immersion handheld blender. Add chicken broth and can of coconut milk, and spices. Heat and cook for 10 minutes on medium. Serve alongside with a fresh salad.

# Simply Healthy Dinners

## TACO SALAD

Tacos are another one of our 'go to' dinners that is well loved by everyone. The kids love assembling their own meal, and we place all the toppings in bowls where they can make their own unique creation. We will rotate between ground grass fed beef, medication free ground turkey or organic quinoa. Serves 4+

### *Ingredients*

½ lb. of grass fed, organic ground meat

Or Vegetarian Option: 2 cups of quinoa & 4 cups water

4 Tbsp. of homemade taco mix (see Spice Mixes) or organic taco seasoning mix.

### *Toppings:*

Chopped fresh tomato

Shredded romaine or chopped spinach

Diced avocado

Diced cilantro

Shredded purple cabbage

Organic salsa

Organic Que Pasa chips or *sweet potato chips

### *Directions*

Fry meat in olive oil till brown, drain the fat, and add seasoning and 1/4 c of water. Cover for 5 minutes.

*To make easy sweet potato chips, simple peel and thinly slice sweet potatoes. Lay flat on a parchment lined cookie tray and bake at 375°F for 20 minutes turning at half time.

For Vegetarian option: Boil water, add quinoa, and simmer, covered, for 15 minutes. Add seasoning to pot of cooked quinoa, stir and transfer to serving dish.

Place everything else in separate bowls for people to create their own meal at the table. Assemble however you like.

# CAMBODIAN CURRY

We do love curry and know it has its benefits as a warming, healing food. You can serve this on a bed of brown rice, or if you are in a hurry, serve on top of brown rice noodles. If you are totally grain free, then you can serve it on top of a bed of raw spinach or heaps of shredded cauliflower (*cauli-rice: shred a head of cauliflower and sauté in pan with 1/3 c of water for 5 minutes till semi-soft). Serves 4+

## *Ingredients*

1-package brown rice vermicelli noodles

2 salmon filets, cut into cubes

1 knob of ginger

4 tbsp quality red or yellow curry paste

1 liter or 5 cups of Organic low sodium vegetable or chicken broth

1 can of full fat coconut milk

3 tbsp fish sauce

2 cups each of chopped broccoli, carrots and red pepper.

1 can of chopped pineapple drained or 1 cup of fresh pineapple

Juice of 1 lime

## *Directions*

Place the rice noodles in a bowl of boiling water and stand for 2 minutes, drain and set aside. If using rice, cook the rice according to package.

Heat up a large wok, or deep pot. Place curry paste and ginger in pot over medium heat and cook for 1 minute. Add the vegetables and cook while coating the vegetables in the paste for about 3-5 minutes. Add broth, fish sauce, lime juice, pineapple, and coconut milk. When the coconut broth is hot (almost boiling), add salmon and cook for 5 minutes. Turn the heat off. Place noodles (or rice or cauliflower 'rice') in bottom of serving bowls and ladle curry over the top. Top with fresh basil if desired.

## SALMON CAKES

This is a staple in our home and highly satisfying all around. It is great with homemade yam fries and a salad. Makes 24 cakes.

### *Ingredients*

3 Cans wild pacific salmon

2 eggs

½ medium onion chopped

1 Tbsp Holy Crap cereal or 1 Tbsp each of Hemp Hearts and Chia Seed

1 tsp each of Comfort Spice mix and Taco Mix OR 1 Tbsp of chutney.

### *Directions*

Mash, beat and combine all ingredients in a medium bowl. Spoon out onto a parchment lined cookie tray as if you are making cookies. Press the cakes down so that they are relatively flat. Bake in oven at 350°F for 20 minutes.

# Favorite Snacks

## DR. J'S FAMOUS POWER MIX

This mix is the most popular request from my family. It is an energy sustaining, protein packable snack that gratifies your body and delights your taste buds. You can make up a few of these and have them at hand for a last minute hike, or after school snack and store them in recycled jam jars. The combination of dried raisins and flakes of dried coconut with beef jerky is sensational.

Note: Nuts and seeds are so filling and super healthy and loaded in iron, calcium, protein, and antioxidants and quality fats. However, try to avoid overconsumption of them as they are also known to have high amounts of phytates, which can contribute to tooth decay and inflammation in the body. I like to borrow a dehydrator once a month and soak and then dehydrate the raw nuts, so that they are neutralized in the body and have a considerably less phytates.

### Ingredients

½ cup of the following combined: pecans

dried raisins or cherries cacao nibs

almonds pumpkin seeds

dried large unsweetened coconut flakes

cut up bits of beef jerky (grass feed, if you can).

*You can substitute the nuts for sunflower seeds for a 'nut free' mix, or add a small handful of quality dark chocolate chips if feel the need for the odd sweet fix-without overdoing it.

# VEGGIE PLATE AND DIPS

One of the tricks I use to ensure my kids get enough veggies is that I serve them about 45 minutes before dinner. I find that just before dinnertime, they have this way of scrounging the kitchen looking for a snack. So, I give them a platter of raw cut veggies and un-hummus, or red pepper/walnut dip which they enjoy so much! Kids have smaller stomachs and therefore their bellies fill up quickly, and that is why kids always seem hungry all the time. They just need smaller meals.

## *Ingredients*

Cut up a variety of raw veggies: carrots, cucumbers, snap peas, red peppers, cherry tomatoes, broccoli, cauliflower and celery. Serve with one of the following dips.

# RED PEPPER WALNUT DIP

## *Ingredients*

> 1 can roasted red peppers, drained
>
> 1 cup roasted walnuts
>
> ½ squeezed lemon
>
> 2 tbsp. chutney or a red fruit jam
>
> 1 crushed garlic clove

## *Directions*

Using a food processor, grind the walnuts first, then add the remaining ingredients for either a dip or a spread.

Both with last for a week stored in a glass jar in the fridge.

# GUACAMOLE

Avocados are a mainstay in our household. Thankfully 3 out of 4 of us love to eat them straight up. However, if you have someone who doesn't like it cut up with a dash of sea salt; you can still get that amazingly health benefits of this super fruit by using it (or disguising it) in a smoothie, chocolate icing, or guacamole.

## *Ingredients*

    1 ripe avocado

    ½ small onion diced

    1 tsp sea salt

    Lemon or lime, optional

## *Directions*

Mash the avocado and stir in the onion and salt. I use an immersion blender and puree all in a bowl. A few squeezes of lime or lemon are a nice addition.


# APPLE OR CELERY SANDIES

Quick and easy and enjoyed by all. Core an apple with apple corer and then make slices so that you have apple rings. Spread almond butter and sprinkle with HolyCrap cereal. You can also dot with a few raisins or dried coconut flakes, and cinnamon. Of course can do the exact same thing with Celery sticks as well and create an upgraded version of 'ants on a log'. (Omit the cinnamon if you are using celery).

# Super Food Treats

## POWER BALL

These are enjoyed as a handy make ahead treat. Great for travel as well. We enjoy eating these anytime knowing we are truly getting a treat packed full of protein, and antioxidants. Makes 12-15 pending on size.

*Ingredients*

½ cup cacao powder (not cocoa powder)

½ cup hemp hearts

½ cup shredded organic unsweetened coconut

½ cup almond butter

2 tablespoons coconut oil

6 dates or 3 tbsp of local honey

1 tsp pure vanilla extract or 1/2 tsp. vanilla powder

*Directions*

Food process if using dates or hand mix in a large mixing bowl if using honey. Roll into small balls and place on cookie sheet lined with parchment paper. Place in the freezer. Once frozen, you can store them in a glass container in the fridge or freezer.

Note: For the Christmas holidays, I stuffed a dried cherry inside the ball. It was a total hit with the entire family and friends, and my son called them "Cherry Bombs". You can also dress these up by rolling them in shredded coconut, dusting them in cacao, or my favorite is to sprinkle coarse Himalayan salt over.

# BAKED APPLES

This has become a really comforting dish for our family, which can be enjoyed for dessert or even breakfast. There is no added sugar, so you will feel pretty balanced and satisfied. Serves 4.

## *Ingredients*

> 4 large apples, cored
>
> 4 tsp coconut oil
>
> ½ cup crumbled pecans
>
> ½ cup raisins
>
> 4 Tbsp cinnamon
>
> 4 medjool dates, pitted

## *Directions*

Set oven to 350°F. Place apples upright in a baking pan (8" x 8"). Mix all ingredients, except apples and dates and then stuff the mixture into the apples. Stuff 1 medjool date in the top and place 1 tbsp. of coconut oil on top and cover in foil. (You can also substitute Weekend Cereal as a stuffing) Bake for 1 hr. Serve warm in individual bowls.

# COCOMACAMATCHA BARS

Don't you just love that say that? Sounds like a latte. These are the king of all power bars and they have high quality fat burning properties and give sustainable energy. The matcha powder is high in antioxidants and boosts your metabolism. The cacao nibs give an added crunch as well as are high in iron. These are one of my favourite go to snacks for that middle of the day drop. You freeze this minty looking mixture and cut them into squares. Enjoy one at a time. Makes 12-15 depending on size.

## *Ingredients*

1 cup unsweetened flaked coconut (60 g)

1 1/2 cups raw, unsalted macadamia nuts (150 to 160 g)

3/4 cup melted coconut oil (180 ml)

1 tablespoon chia seeds (15 ml)

2 TBSP of BP Collagen

1 TSP macha powder

1/3 c cacao nibs

Pinch of sea salt

## *Directions*

Preheat oven to 350 °F.

Put the coconut flakes in a pan and toast in the oven until lightly browned, about five minutes.

Line an 8×8 pan with parchment paper.

Process the macadamia nuts, coconut oil, collagen, and macha powder in a food processor until very smooth. Add the coconut flakes and chia seeds and pulse a few times. Stir in the cacao nibs.

Pour the batter into the 8×8 pan. Sprinkle a pinch of sea salt on top

# Essential Time Savers

It can be so frustrating when you have full intentions to make healthy meals for the rest of your life and then find yourself overwhelmed with all the prep work and clean up. It is those times that you can be very vulnerable and default to take out, or giving up on the entire healthy eating process entirely. Don't worry, I've been there. After many failed initial attempts and false starts, here are a few time saver tips that are proven to be very effective.

## TIME SAVER TIPS

1. **Boil a few eggs** and store in fridge for up to a week. Instant protein, packable and perfect addition to any salad.

2. **Make turkey meatballs and freeze**. Drop directly into a hot cooking tomato pasta sauce or soup. Reheat in oven for afterschool snacks or lunches.

3. **Buy your organic lettuce pre-washed and ready**. In the wintertime, I splurge and buy the cartons of organic pre-washed spinach or mixed lettuce. It's easy to make a quick salad, or add to boost your stews or soups, or omelets.

4. **Make salmon cakes and freeze.** Reheat in oven. Perfect for all meals alone with roasted vegetables, or on top a salad. Can add to squash soup base to create a fabulous salmon chowder.

5. **Double soup recipes and freeze in ice cube trays.** Then put into freezer bags so that you can take what you need to add to curries, stews, and soups.

6. **Meal Plan** once a week and stick to the grocery list.

7. **Mix spice mixes and dressings in advance.** Spices can be made once a month and dressings can be made at the beginning of the week.

8. **Make granola and porridge mix ahead** of time and store in jar in fridge.

9. **Leftover cooked chicken breast meat can be cut into cubes** and stored in a freezer bag. Add frozen to soups, or defrost to add to a salad or create a chicken kebab with cherry tomatoes for the kids' lunch.

10. **Get to know your crockpot.** So nice to come home during a busy work week and not have to start preparing a meal. The smell of a hearty stew or soup piping through the kitchen is strangely calming. There are many amazing blogs to find healthy crockpot stews and soups, which are listed under the Resources section.

# The Grand Finale

*"Life is no brief candle to me. It is a sort of splendid torch which I have got a hold of for the moment, and I want to make it burn as brightly as possible before handing it on to future generations."*
-George Bernard Shaw

Many people have well-meaning intentions to make a change in their lives, but just don't know how to begin. Now after reading this book, you have the How, What, When and Where. But even if you have all the knowledge now, I can assure you that nothing will be sustainable unless you have the "Why".

Your Why!

Your "why" needs to be anchored in your heart in order to make changes and have them stick. Your WHY needs to be bigger than you.

Start with asking yourself *"What is it that makes you want to even consider changing?"* Write your answer down. You don't need to complicate it. It is simply already in you. Just get it out. Write it down here. You don't need a fancy piece of paper. Just write out what is flowing from your heart. On the next page, there is a simple process to help 'Discover Your Why'.

At the end of every workshop I ask the question "Why do you want to be healthy?" Many people say, "So I can be happy". Others will say, "So I can be fit." Or simply others will sit in silence pondering that question. I challenge you to ponder that question more. Because ultimately,

"what is the number one thing most important to you?"

Your health?

True, and I would agree.

AND... I would ask again, "Ok, then why do you want to be healthy?"

And after some contemplation and digging deep, I'm certain you will agree that the answer in its simplicity, is the essence of what you are created for:

'love'

love

love

love

## — to Love and Be Loved!

So to me, health is number two; love is number one.

Simply put, be healthy and fully alive, so you can be present and serve the people you love. I truly believe God loves you and has great plans for you. I hope that this inspires you to find your big WHY.

*If I speak in the tongues of men or of angels,
but do not have love, I am only a resounding
gong or a clanging cymbal. If I have the gift
of prophecy and can fathom all mysteries and
all knowledge, and if I have a faith that can
move mountains, but do not have love, I am
nothing. If I give all I possess to the poor and
give over my body to hardship that I may
boast, but do not have love, I gain nothing.*

*Love is patient, love is kind. It does not envy,
it does not boast, it is not proud. It does not
dishonor others, it is not self-seeking, it is not
easily angered, it keeps no record of wrongs.
Love does not delight in evil but rejoices with
the truth. It always protects, always trusts,
always hopes, always perseveres.*

*Love never fails.*

*1 Corrinthians 13: 1-8*

# Discover Your Why!

*Read the following declarations out loud as you fill in the blanks.*

I want to be healthy so that I...

_____(A)

And if I could ...

*(Insert your
answer from A here)*_____

I would ...

_____(B)

**Digging Deeper:** What would B do for you?

And if I...

*(Insert your
answer from B here)*_____

I would...

_____(Your Why)

# Resources

I am constantly reviewing new websites, blogs, books and apps. Follow me at DrJodyCox.com to check out what I am learning. For now, these are solid resources.


## RECOMMENDED WEBSITES

Drjodycox.com

Chiropractors with Compassion – www.cwc.org

International Chiropractic Pediatric Association for Kids – icpa4kids.com

Healthy Child Healthy World – healthychild.org

Female Pelvic Floor Care – Femfusionfitness.com

Ideal Spine –idealspine.com

Dr. Mercola – mercola.com

Whole9 –whole9life.com

Chiropractic: Torquerelease.ca

12 Minute Workout - HIITit.ca (visit my website for a promo code.)

Bees and Honey - Robertscreekhoney.com

Bullet Proof – bulletproof.com

Drpompa.com

# RECOMMENDED BLOGS

My New Roots: mynewroots.org

If Gathering: ifgathering.com

Detoxinista: detoxinista.com

Nom Nom Paleo: nomnompaleo.com

# RECOMMENDED FREE APPS

Seven: no gym required workout that you can use literally anywhere anytime and will work every part of your body for literally 7 minutes.

Elevation Network or Fresh Life Church: instant access to biblically sound inspiring messages

Nike + Fitness App (free): simple to use and track your running pace, time and distance while running or jogging.

Spine Design: detailed anatomy to give a reference to any part of the spine and how it works synergistically with associated nerves, muscles and ligaments.

# RECOMMENDED BOOKS

*Well Adjusted Babies* – Dr. Jennifer Barham-Floreani

*Marathoning for Mortals* –John Bingham& Jennie Hadfield

*Willing to Walk on Water* – Caroline Barnett

*The Gift in You* - Caroline Leaf

*One Thousand Gifts*—Ann Voskamp

*Through the Eyes of a Lion* – Levi Lusko

*Greater & Crash the Chatterbox*–Steven Furdick

*It Starts with Food* – Dallas & Melissa Hartwig

*Grain Brain* – David Perlmutter

*Against All Grain* - Danielle Walker

*Meals Made Simply* & *Celebrations* - Danielle Walker

*Oh She Glows* – Angela Liddon

*The Simply Raw Kitchen* – Natasha Kyssa

*Love Does* – Bob Goth

*The Power of Positive Thinking* - Vincent Pearle

*The Green Smoothie Bible* – Kristine Miles

*The Performance Paleo Cookbook* – Stephanie Gaudreau

*The Bank on Yourself Revolution* – Pamela Yellen

# About The Author

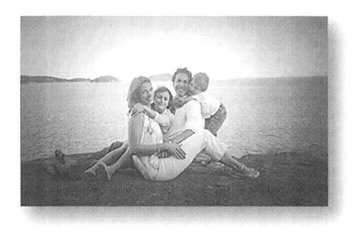

Dr. Jody Cox, DC

I am a wife, mother, Chiropractor, friend and sports enthusiast. I am a regular person following my calling to bring new hope to people in any way I can, but mainly through the gift and practice of chiropractic.

Over the past two decades of practice, training around the world, mission trips to Africa, and professional and personal coaching, I have learnt (and am still learning) that true health comes from above-down-inside-out (not outside in). That chiropractic is a lifestyle choice focused on creating health, not treating disease. That the choices you make today, right now, can transform your life for years to come.

I absolutely LOVE adjusting people and can't believe I get the privilege of serving people everyday. I have witnessed hundreds of people go...

...From despair to hopeful

...From grumpy to joyful

...From suffering from debilitating pain to being able to finally go ski down a mountain with their family

I get to watch kids who were once deemed to be asthmatic for the rest of their lives, to playing soccer and running –asthma free.

..all through the living principles of chiropractic.

Here is what I believe:

I believe everybody – including kids, is designed and create to be healthy-from Above Down Inside Out. And not just escaping with drugs for chronic stressors but living an unprocessed life to the point where you are smiling from within, so that you can fully express who you truly are and live out your God given purpose while here on earth.

As a family chiropractor who is passionate about taking care of kids and leading families to be fully alive through the principles of Chiropractic, I get the privilege to adjust people's spines.

And by change the physiology in your spine and nervous system, it changes the physiology in your health-for the better. So you can do what you *need* to do with ease and do what you *Love* to do with abundant energy.

The Best is Yet to Come!

Dr.JODY

## PARTIAL PROCEEDS FROM THIS BOOK GO TO CHIROPRACTORS WITH COMPASSION.

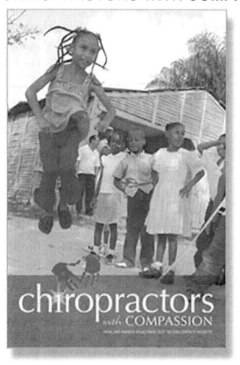

## HEALING HANDS REACHING OUT TO CHILDREN'S HEARTS

Chiropractors with Compassion (CWC) is a movement dedicated to transforming the lives of children around the world. Chiropractors from around North America have joined hands together with Compassion to fund holistic child centered projects around the globe.

Each project is focused on transforming children from the inside-out by serving their spiritual, educational, economic, social and physical needs.

By focusing on *developing* the child, we help break the cycle of poverty.

We believe that these children have the potential not only to survive, but to thrive; to become leaders in their community who will in turn bring change to the world around them.

Every project is funded by CWC doctors, who have each committed to donate $20 from every new patient exam.

CWC is bringing help and hope to impoverished children and is allowing the hearts of individual chiropractors to grow as they serve and give to those in need.

Chiropractors of all practice philosophies and styles are coming together to serve children in a tangible way.

Healing hands have joined together to transform the world one child at a time and we're just getting started... Chiropractors with Compassion is a partner with Compassion Canada.

# Endnotes

[1] Chronic Disease Surveillance and Monitoring Division, CCDP, Public Health Agency of Canada. Canadian Cancer Society. 2013.

[2] *Causes of Death 1992* (Ministry of Industry, Science and Technology, Statistics Canada, Health Statistics Division, Sept. 1994); and, *Method of Committing Homicide Offences, Canadian the Provinces/Territories, 1992* (Ministry of Industry, Science and Technology, Statistics Canada, Canadian Centre for Justice Statistics, 1992)

[3] http://healthycanadians.gc.ca

[4] *Causes of Death 1992* (Ministry of Industry, Science and Technology, Statistics Canada, Health Statistics Division, Sept. 1994); and, *Method of Committing Homicide Offences, Canadian the Provinces/Territories, 1992* (Ministry of Industry, Science and Technology, Statistics Canada, Canadian Centre for Justice Statistics, 1992)

[5] Journal American Medical Association July 26, 2000;284(4):483-5

[6] New appreciation of serious adverse drug reactions Issue: BCMJ, Vol. 47, No. 1, January, February 2005, page(s) 14 BC Centre for Disease Control Barbara Cadario, BSc, BScPhm, MSc

[7] Baker G, Norton P, Flintoff V, et al. The Canadian adverse events study: The incidence of adverse events among hospital patients in

Canada. CMAJ 2004; 170: 1678-86.

Canadian Institute for Health Information. (2004). Health care in Canada. CIHI: Ottawa; 2004: 16-22.

Medical Error in Canada: Issues Related to Reporting of Medical Error and Methods to Increase Reporting. Atif R. Butt, BA, MBA, CHE Clinical Review: Volume 7 No. 1, 2010

[8] Department of Health and Human Services. January 2012 OEI-06-09-00091

[9] World Health Report 2000. Accessed June 28, 2000.

[10] Holy Bible. English Standard Version. Genesis 2:7 – *then the LORD God formed the man of dust from the ground and breathed into his nostrils the breath of life, and the man became a living creature.*

[11] Holy Bible, English Standard Version. Ezekiel 37: 4-5 *Then he said to me, "Prophesy over these bones, and say to them , O dry bones, hear the word of the LORD. Thus says the LORD GOD to these bones: Behold, I will cause breath to enter you, and you shall live."*

[12] Holy Bible, English Standard Version. Job 33:4 *The Spirit of God had made me, and the breath of the Almighty gives me life.*

[13] Breig, Alf. Adverse Mechanical Tension in the Central Nervous System: An Analysis of Cause and Effect. 1978. Almqvuist & Wiksell International, Stockholm,Sweden. Pg. 177.

[14] Towbin A. Latent spinal cord and brain stem injury in newborn infants. Dev Med Child Neurol. 1969 Feb;11(1):54-68.

[15] Pettibon, Burl, DC and Hawkins-Hals , Jenn. Aricles on HeadForward and Antalgic Postures are Accumulative Injuries. www.info.pettibonsystem.com/psoas-stretch fulcrum.

[16] *Spine*, 1986;6:591-694

[17] 31st Annual International Conference of the IEEE EMBS Minneapolis, Minnesota, USA, September 2-6, 2009

[18] Breig, Alf. Adverse Mechanical Tension in the Central Nervous System: An Analysis of Cause and Effect. 1978. Almqvuist & Wiksell International, Stockholm, Sweden. Pg. 177

[19] Henry Windsor, MD, published in the Medical Times 1921, Sympathetic Segmental Dysfunction and Visceral Pathology. Reviewing the work of Henry Windsor, Dan Murphy, American Journal of Clinical Chiropractic, July 2004.

[20] Korr IM. The spinal cord as organizer of disease processes. J AM Osteopath Association. 1976; Sept; 76(1) 35-45

[21] (Mayo Clinic Health, March 2000).

[22] (Cephalgia, February 2009).

[23] Cailliet R, Gross L, Rejuvenation Strategy. New York, Doubleday and Co. 1987

[24] (Kapandji, Phys of Joints Vol. 3).

[25] (Dr. Alf Breig, Neurosurgeon and Nobel Prize Recipient).

[26] Sperry, R. W. (1988) Roger Sperry's brain research. Bulletin of The Theosophy Science Study Group 26(3-4), 27-28. Nerve Connections. Quart. Rev. Biol. 46, 198

[27] (Rene Cailliet, Improvement in Forward Head Posture, Cervical Lordosis, and Pulmonary Function with Chiropractic Care, Anterior Head Weighting and Whole Body Vibration: A Retrospective Study-Mark Morningstar DC, DAASP, FRCCM, FAAIM 1, David Jockers DC, MS, CSCS2J. Pediatric, Maternal & Family Health - October 12, 2009)

[28] Cailliet R, Gross L, Rejuvenation Strategy. New York, Doubleday and Co. 1987

[29] Harrison DD, Jackson BL, Troyanovich SJ, Robertson GA, DeGeorge D, Barker WF. The Efficacy of Cervical Extension-Compression Traction Combined with Diversified Manipulation and Drop Table Adjustments in the Rehabilitation of Cervical Lordosis. J Manipulative Physiol Ther 1994;17(7):454-464.

[30] Retrospective Birth Dating of Cells in Humans. Kirsty L. Spalding, Ratan D. Bhardwaj, Bruce A. Buchholz, Henrik Druid, and Jonas Frisén. Cell, Vol 122, 133-143, 15 July 2005

[31] Korr IM. The spinal cord as organizer of disease processes. J AM Osteopath Association. 1976; Sept; 76(1) 35-45

[32] Harrison, K. L. (1979). "Fetal Erythrocyte Lifespan". Journal of Paediatrics and Child Health 15 (2): 96–97.

[33] Harrison DE, Cailliet R, Harrison DD, Janik TJ, Holland B. New 3-Point Bending Traction Method of Restoring Cervical Lordosis Combined with Cervical Manipulation: Non-randomized Clinical Control Trial. Arch Phys Med Rehab 2002; 83(4): 447-453.

[34] http://articles.mercola.com/sites/articles/archive/2005/06/11/spinal- regeneration.aspx

[35] Chestnut, J.L. 2003 The 14 Foundational Premises for the Scientific and Philosophical Validation of the Chiropractic Wellness Paradigm. Pg. 222

[36] British Journal of Sports Medicine. 2013-093342. Sept 2014. Per Sjogren, Rachel Fisher, Lena Kallings, Ulrika Svenson, Goran Roos, Mai-Lis Hellenius. Stand up for health-avoiding sedentary behavior might lengthen your telomeres: secondary outcomes from a physical activity RCT in older people.

[37] Sedentary behavior and life expectancy in the USA: a cause-

deleted life table analysis. Katzmarzyk PT, Lee IM. BMJ Open. 2012 Jul 9; 2(4). pii: e000828.

38 Standing and mortality in a prospective cohort of Canadian adults. Katzmarzyk PT., Med Sci Sports Exerc. 2014 May;46(5):940-6

39 Heydari, M., Freund, J., & Boutcher, S. H. (2012). The Effect of High-Intensity Intermittent Exercise on Body Composition of Overweight Young Males. *Journal of Obesity, 2012*

40 Trapp EG, Chisholm DJ, Freund J, Boutcher SH. The effects of high-intensity intermittent exercise training on fat loss and fasting insulin levels of young women. *International Journal of Obesity.* 2008;32(4):684–691

41 Adapted from Mercola.com

42 Henry Windsor, MD, published in the Medical Times 1921, Sympathetic Segmental Dysfunction and Visceral Pathology. Reviewing the work of Henry Windsor, Dan Murphy, American Journal of Clinical Chiropractic, July 2004.

43 Curtis Fedorchuk DC and Andrew St. Bernard DC. Improvement in Gastro Esophageal Reflux Disease Following Chiropractic Care and the ALCAT Procedure. Annals of Vertebral Subluxation Research, June 23, 2011, pp 44-50.

44 Chronic Disease State Policy Tracking System. Date accessed June 1, 2012. Available at *http://apps.nccd.cdc.gov/CDPHPPolicySearch.*

45 Mercola.com

46 *Nourishing Traditions. Sally Fallon, New Trends Publishing, Inc. 2001

47 Grain Brain, David Pearlmutter.

48 Mercola.com/brain facts.

[49] It's Starts With Food. Dallas and Mellisa Hartwig. Victory Belt Publishing. 2012

[50] Daley, C., Abbott, A., Doyle., P. et al. (2010). A review of fatty acid profiles and antioxidant content in grass-fed and grain-fed beef. *Nutrition Journal, 9*:10.

[51] Lenoir M, Serre F, Cantin L, Ahmed SH (2007) Intense Sweetness Surpasses Cocaine Reward. PLoS ONE 2(8): e698. doi:10.1371/journal.pone.0000698

[52] American Society for Microbiology. "Humans Have Ten Times More Bacteria Than Human Cells: How Do Microbial Communities Affect Human Health?" ScienceDaily. ScienceDaily, 5 June 2008.

[53] Burgess, John R., et al. Long-chain polyunsaturated fatty acids in children with attention-deficit hyperactivity disorder. American Journal of Clinical Nutrition, Vol. 71 (suppl), January 2000, pp. 327S

[54] Stoll, Andrew L., et al. Omega 3 fatty acids in bipolar disorder. Archives of General Psychiatry, Vol. 56, May 1999, pp. 407-12 and pp. 415-16.

[55] Metabolic syndrome' in the brain: deficiency in omega-3 fatty acid exacerbates dysfunctions in insulin receptor signaling and cognition Rahul Agrawal[1] and Fernando Gomez-Pinilla[1,2] The Journal of Physiology. Volume 590, Issue 10, pages 2485–2499, May 2012

[56] How Much Vitamin D Do You Really Need to Take? Mercola.com /Vitamin D

[57] *Ann of Epidemiology*, 2009

[58] Batmanghelidj, F.: Your Body's Many Cries for Water. Global Health Solutions, Inc. 2008 p. 14-15

[59] Amha Belay, Yoshimichi Ota (1993): Current knowledge on potential health benefits of Spirulina. Pub. in Journal of Appl.

Phycology, 5:235-241.

[60] http://www.ewg.org/foodnews/methodology.php

[61] Bouchard M, Bellinger D, Wright R, Weisskopf M. 2010. Attention-Deficit/Hyperactivity Disorder and Urinary Metabolites of Organophosphate Pesticides. Pediatrics 125: 1270-77.

[62] CDC (U.S. Centers for Disease Control and Prevention). 2009b. Fourth National Report on Human Exposure to Environmental Chemicals. Department of Health and Human Services

[63] Concept inspired from our friends, the Wiebe family and www.summitchiropractic.ca

[64] Lucassen EA, Piaggi P, Dsurney J, de Jonge L, Zhao X-c, et al. (2014) Sleep Extension Improves Neurocognitive Functions in Chronically Sleep- Deprived Obese Individuals. PLoS ONE 9(1): e84832. doi:10.1371/journal.pone.0084832

[65] Castro, J. "Sleep's Secret Repairs." *Scientific American Mind* 23, No. 2 (2012): 42- 45.

[66] Brain Rules: 12 Principles for Surviving and Thriving at Work, Home, and School; John Medina. Pear Press | March 10, 2009

[67] National Institutes of Health. National Sleep Foundation.

[68] Walker MP. Cognitive consequences of sleep and sleep loss. Sleep Medicine 2008; 16(5): 287-298.

[69] Onen SH1, Onen F, Bailly D, Parquet P. Prevention and treatment of sleep disorders through regulation] of sleeping habits. Presse Med. 1994 Mar 12;23(10):485-9. [70] Joyce Miller, Joyce D.C., F.A.C.O., F.C.C. and Matts, Klemsdal, Matts. Can chiropractic care improve infants' Sleep? Journal of Clinical Chiropractic Pediatrics. Volume 9, Number 1. March 2008

[71] "thanks" , How the New Science of Gratitude Can make you

Happier, by Robert Emmons

[72] Purcell, M. (2006). The Health Benefits of Journaling. *Psych Central.* Retrieved on February 4, 2015, from http://psychcentral.com/lib/the-health-benefits-of-journaling/000721

[73] Vancouver study: A city of loneliness and unfriendliness? Local survey also finds gaps between ethnic and linguistic communities by Craig Takeuchi on June 19th, 2012

[74] Doidge, Norman, MD. The Brain That Changes Itself: Stories of Personal Triumph from the Frontiers of Brain Science

[75] Kenfield, S.A. *The Journal of the American Medical Association,* May 7, 2008; vol 299: pp 2037-2047.

[76] Cerebral metabolic changes after chiropractic spinal manipulation. Alternative Therapies Health Medicine. 2011 Nov-Dec; 17 (6): 12-7

[77] Coulter ID, Hurwitz EL, Aronow HU, et al: "Chiropractic patients in a comprehensive home-based geriatric assessment, follow-up and health promotion program." Topics in Clinical Chiropractic 1996;3(2):46.

[78] Rupert RL, Manello D, Sandefur R: "Maintenance care: Health promotion services administered to U.S. chiropractic patients aged 65 or older, Part II." Journal of Manipulative and Physiological Therapeutics 2000;23(1):10.

[79] Blanks RHI, Schuster TL, Dobson M: "A retrospective assessment of network care using a survey of self- reported health, wellness and quality of life." Journal of Vertebral Subluxation Research 1997;1(4):15.

[80] Sarnat RL, Winterstein J, Cambron JA: "Clinical utilization and cost outcomes from an integrative medicine independent physician association: an additional 3-year update." J Manipulative Physiol Ther 2007;30(4):263-269.

[81] Hyper Kyphotic posture predicts mortality in older community-dwelling men and women. J AM Geriatric Soc. 2004 Oct; 52(10): 1662-7

[82] Fast A. Low Back Pain in Pregnancy. Spine. 1987; 12 (4); 368-371

[83] Lisi, Anthony J. Chiropractic Spinal Manipulation for Low Back Pain of Pregnancy: a retrospective case series. Journal of Midwifery Womens Health 2006 (Jan);51)1): e7-10.

[84] J.M. Fallon. Textbook on chiropractic & pregnancy.

Arlington, VA: International Chiropractic Association; 1994: 52, 109.

[85] Thompson CK. Baby on board: the benefit of chiropractic during pregnancy for both mother and child. J Am Chiropr Assoc 1997; 34(5):17, 95

[86] The Webster Technique: a chiropractic technique with obstetric implications. *Pistolese RA. J Manipulative Physiol Ther. 2002 Jul-Aug; 25(6):E1-9.*

[87] Towbin A. Latent spinal cord and brain stem injuries in newborn infants. Develop Med Child Neurol. 1969; 11, 54-68

[88] Biedermann H. Kinematic imbalances due to subocciptal strain in newborns. J Manual Med. 1992 6:151-156

[89] Chestnut J DC. The 14 Foundational Premises for the Scientific and Philosophical Validation for the Chiropractic Wellness Paradigm. Canada: Chestnut Wellness and Chiropractic Corporation: 2003

[90] Towbin A. Latent spinal cord and brain stem injury in newborn infants. Develp Med Child Neorol 1969; 11:54-

68 Birth trauma causes spinal injury. The effect is lifelong impairment

[91] van Breda WM. Van Breda JM. A comparative Study of the Health Status of Children Riased under the Health models of

Chiropractic and Allopathic medicine. J Chiro Research. 1989: 101-103

92 Lewit K. Barth JA Leipzig. Functional Disorders of the Spine in Children. Maneulle Therapie. 1973; 2 (7): 50-54.

93 van Breda WM. Van Breda JM. A comparative Study of the Health Status of Children Riased under the Health models of Chiropractic and Allopathic medicine. J Chiro Research. 1989: 101-103

94 McMullen M. Physical stresses of childhood that could lead to need for chiropractic care. ICA International Review of Chiropractic. 1995; 51 (1): 24-28

95 Biedermann H. Kinematic imbalances due to subocciptal strain in newborns. J Manual Med. 1992 6:151-156

96 Journal of Manipulative & Physiological Therapeutics August 1989

97 J Manipulative Physiol Ther. 1996 Mar- Apr;19(3):169-77. Ear infection: a retrospective study examining improvement from chiropractic care and analyzing for influencing factors. Froehle RM.

98 Haavik Taylor, H and Murphy B.A. (2007) Cervical spine manipulation alters sensorimotor integration: a somatosensory evoked potential study. J of Clinical Neurophysiology, 118(2): 391-402.

99 SOURCES: Legorreta, A.P. *Archives of Internal Medicine*, Oct. 11, 2004; vol 164: pp 1985-1992. Douglas Metz, DC, chief health services officer, American Specialty Health Plans, San Diego. George DeVries, president and CEO, American Specialty Health Plans, San Diego. Scott Boden, MD, professor of orthopaedics, Emory University School of Medicine; director, Emory Orthopaedic and Spine Center, Atlanta.

[100] Campbell CJ, Kent C, Banne A, Amri A, Per R. Surrogate Indication of DNA Repair in Serum After Long Term Chiropractic Intervention0a Retrospective study. JVSR. 2005. (pg 1-5)

[101] Pero R. Cited in: Rosso J. (2004) Boosting Immunity through chiro-practic. Available: www.bizmonthly.com/6 1998focus/delross.html.

[102] Campbell CJ, Kent C, Banne A, Amri A, Per R. Surrogate Indication of DNA Repair in Serum After Long Term Chiropractic Intervention Retrospective study. JVSR. 2005. (pg 1-5)

[103] Atlas vertebra realignment and achievement of arterial pressure goal in hypertensive patients. Journal of Human Hypertension. 2007 21: 347-352.

[104] Innocuous mechanical stimulation of the neck and alterations in heart-rate variability in healthy young adults. Auton Neuroscience, 2001 Aug 13;91(1-2):96-9

[105] Measurable Changes in the neuro-endocrinal mechanism following spinal manipulation. Journal of Medical Hypotheses (2015).

[106] Vector. 1999;2(4).

[107] JMPT 2007

[108] Cailliet R, Gross L, Rejuvenation Strategy. New York, Doubleday and Co. 1987

[109] The effects of Specific Upper Cervical Adjustments on the CD4 Counts of HIV-Positive Patients, Selano, Highwater et al. The Chiro. Research Journal, 3(1), 1994

Made in the USA
San Bernardino, CA
09 September 2018